Time as a Factor in Groupwork: Time-Limited Group Experiences

The *Social Work with Groups* series

Series Editors: Catherine P. Papell and Beulah Rothman

- *Co-Leadership in Social Work with Groups*, Catherine P. Papell and Beulah Rothman

- *Social Groupwork & Alcoholism*, Marjorie Altman and Ruth Crocker, Guest Editors

- *Groupwork with the Frail Elderly*, Shura Saul, Guest Editor

- *The Use of Group Services in Permanency Planning for Children*, Sylvia Morris, Guest Editor

- *Activities and Action in Groupwork,* Ruth Middleman, Guest Editor

- *Groupwork with Women/Groupwork with Men: An Overview of Gender Issues in Social Groupwork Practice*, Beth Glover Reed and Charles D. Garvin, Guest Editors

- *Ethnicity in Social Group Work Practice*, Larry Davis, Guest Editor

- *Groupwork with Children and Adolescents,* Ralph Kolodny and James Garland, Guest Editors

- *Time as a Factor in Groupwork: Time-Limited Group Experiences*, Albert S. Alissi and Max Casper, Guest Editors

- *William Schwartz Memorial Issue* (title to be announced), Alex Gitterman and Lawrence Shulman, Guest Editors

- *Research in Group Work,* Ronald A. Feldman, Guest Editor; Larry E. Davis, Maeda Galinsky, Sheldon D. Rose, Martin Sundel, James K. Whittaker, Associate Guest Editors

- *Effectiveness in Service Delivery: Administrative Groups*, Ronald Toseland and Paul Ephross, Guest Editors

- *The Concept of Collectivity: Operationalizing Theory*, Norma C. Lang, Guest Editor

Time as a Factor in Groupwork: Time-Limited Group Experiences

Albert S. Alissi and Max Casper
Guest Editors

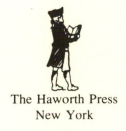

The Haworth Press
New York

Time as a Factor in Groupwork: Time-Limited Group Experiences has also been published as *Social Work with Groups,* Volume 8, Number 2, Summer 1985.

The Haworth Press, Inc., 28 East 22 Street, New York, NY 10010

Library of Congress Cataloging in Publication Data
Main entry under title:

Time as a factor in groupwork.

    Bibliography: p.
    1. Social group work—Addresses, essays, lectures.
I. Alissi, Albert S.   II. Casper, Max.   III. Title: Time-limited group experiences.
HV45.T57   1985   361.4   85-7636
ISBN 0-86656-409-8
ISBN 0-86656-438-1 (pbk.)

Time as a Factor in Groupwork: Time-Limited Group Experiences

Social Work with Groups
Volume 8, Number 2

CONTENTS

EDITORIAL   1

GUEST EDITORIAL: Time as a Factor in Social
  Groupwork   3
            Albert S. Alissi
            Max Casper

Time-Limited Treatment Groups for Children   17
            Steven R. Rose

Transition to Parenthood: A Time-Limited Mutual
  Aid Group to Facilitate a Major Role Change   29
            Nancy Boyd Webb

The Neighborhood Group: A Reminiscence Group
  for the Disoriented Old   43
            Lorrie Greenhouse Gardella

When Time Counts: Poetry and Music in Short-Term
  Group Treatment   53
            Nicholas Mazza
            Barbara D. Price

Patterns of Entry and Exit in Open-Ended Groups   67
            Maeda J. Galinsky
            Janice H. Schopler

On the Potentiality and Limits of Time: The
  Single-Session Group and the Cancer Patient   81
            Lisa Rae Block

Children's Single-Session Briefings: Group Work
with Military Families Experiencing Parents'
Deployment   101
    Jane A. Waldron
    Ronaele R. Whittington
    Steve Jensen

A Behavioral Approach to Time-Limited Groups   111
    Martin Sundel
    Sandra Stone Sundel

PRACTICE NOTES

Aerobic Therapy: A Feminist/Wholistic Approach
in Time-Limited Group Practice   125
    Nan Van Den Bergh

Administrative Assistants in the Public School:
The Underutilized Resource   130
    Andrew Malekoff
    Martin Golloub

Bridging the Isolation Gap: Making a Telephone
Connection   134
    Ruth Pollock Shilman
    Beth Horowitz Giladi

An Eclectic Approach to Group Work with the
Alcoholic's "Family" System During Short-Term
Inpatient Treatment   137
    David J. Matulis

Effects of Time Limitation in a Low Self-Concept
Children's Group   139
    Barry M. Daste
    Patricia O. Cox

The Single Session Group: An Innovative Approach
to the Waiting Room   143
    Tryna Rotholz

Characteristics and Consequences of a Time-Limited
Writing Group in an Academic Setting   146
    Kathleen J. Pottick
    Anne Currin Adams
    Audrey Olsen Faulkner

Time Limited Training for Group Leadership   149
    Barbara Dazzo

Practice Quiz: Recurring Issues in Working with
Time Limited Groups: Four Vignettes   151
    Joe Lassner

An Ego-Oriented, Goal-Directed, Short-Term Treatment
Model of Groupwork with Cancer Patients and Their
Families   154
    Sarajane P. McNulty Schaefer

The "Caring for Your Aging Parent" Group   157
    Connie Morse McCaffrey

Time as a Factor in Groupwork: Time-Limited Group Experiences

EDITORIAL

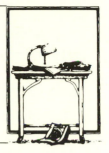

The Editors of *Social Work with Groups* submit this issue to our readers in recognition of the universal interest and concern of the human services in Time as a significant variable.

In the work of the helping professions Time has moved into the consciousness of recipients as well as providers of service. Whether Time is conceived as boundary, process, technique or constraint, there can be no timeless practice. Closure is a built-in expectancy from the out-set in contemporary practice, more often now made explicit as a condition of service by client and worker.

The rapidity of movement of our modern world—in production, communication, problem-solving—renders Time a scarce resource. The juxtaposed advantages of the computer with the potential destructiveness of nuclear weapons places Time in the center of every person's awareness, carrying with it a challenging possibility as well as ominous forboding.

Post industrial society equates Time with efficiency. Our guest editors, however, keep us on balance as professionals. In this issue they view Time in terms of effectiveness of service and sensitivity to the human condition. For this we are grateful to them and we are appreciative of their leadership and creativity in making this volume possible.

CPP
BR

GUEST EDITORIAL

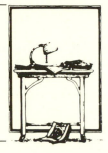

Time as a Factor in Social Groupwork

The purpose of this special issue of *Social Work with Groups* is to alert the reader to regard time as a variable that can be used consciously with groups to help people help themselves. The underlying premise is that the time-limited group can provide the leverage to enrich the outcomes of group experience. We therefore offer here an historical perspective on time-limited groups, a framework for their analysis, and a glimpse of time as the context for effective change.

> Please do not take me for granted! I have limited existence. I can have many purposes. I can benefit you, your colleagues, your family, your clients. In return, I need your willingness to listen, to look. I invite you to budget and invest a wee bit of your time. I encourage you to risk some of your energy and share your personal expertise in a potentially useable experi-

Albert S. Alissi, DSW, MSSA is Professor of Social Work, University of Connecticut, Greater Hartford Campus, West Hartford, Connecticut 06117. Max Casper, ACSW is Associate Professor, Syracuse University School of Social Work, Brockway Hall, Syracuse, New York 13210.

ence. Who am I? Today, I am a time-limited group. (Casper, 1983)

Among the more exciting developments for those of us identified with social group work over the years, has been the recognition by others that there really is a power in the small group experience that can be tapped to help people. This is evidenced in the introduction of group methods into virtually every aspect of social work practice. It is also reflected in the rapid proliferation of comparable group methods within the various disciplines which have spawned divergent views regarding the benefits to be gained from one or another kind of group experience. Increasingly, attention is focussed on one or another factor such as age, gender, co-leadership, programming, to assess its impact on practice. This special edition highlights the conscious use of time as a strategic variable in social work with groups and addresses the ways in which time-limited group experiences are used to carry out varied social work goals and objectives.

We are accustomed to the idea that special editions such as this that deal with selective facets of practice will somehow pull together loose ends in our thinking and at the very least summarize the current state of the art concerning those practices. Implied is the expectation that new ground will be broken and that an exciting new course of action will set forth that will set a trend of significant things to come. If this is what readers will be looking for here, we must warn them from the start that these expectations were only partially, if at all, accomplished in this compilation. We make no excuses except to say that they will find, as we did, that there were indeed many loose ends to be pulled together. Reports from the field are encouraging, but—as is true in much of what we do—there was a scarcity of "hard" data comparing methods and linking them to outcomes. Moreover, there were the usual definitional and conceptual ambiguities concerning the essential elements underlying time-limited group methods. Consistent with the time-limited themes discussed herein, the reader is urged to scale down expectations, specify his or her goals, structure reading time to do what is do-able, and above all, regard the experience as only the beginning of still better things to come.

Contrary to what some might think, time-limited group work is not foreign to social group workers who have traditionally stressed the myriad powers that reside in varied group experiences. To be sure, early group workers often talked about "group living" which conveyed their sense of pervasiveness of small group experience as an on-going phenomena. Groups were endemic; and, one kind of practice in particular—social group work—has a profound influence on its members in helping them grow and develop, in resolving interpersonal problems, preventing social breakdown, inculcating democratic values, fostering social responsibility, and so on. Moyle (1946), for example, writing in *The Group*, distinguished between the comparatively short-term relationships identified with psychiatric and casework services from the "long-term participation" of the "developmental type" identified with group work. The social group work process was clearly a process of "becoming" which was long and arduous.

But, as a practical matter, groups functioned under the usual time constraints placed on people living in complex societies. Wilson and Ryland (1949) for example, talked about helping group members budget time as they did money. "Time," they pointed out, "is a real factor which must be reckoned with in all of life, and the worker who helps the members to use its limitations effectively is helping them learn an important element in successful living" (p. 168). In a more deliberate use of time, Louise Shoemaker (1960) urged group workers to learn how to "accelerate the group processes" to help groups move at a pace that was realistic and possible. The transitory nature of short-term groups did not, in her view, detract in any away from what might be possible in the longer-term group experiences. In either case, members were to be helped to mobilize their strengths in using present experiences in the group to become more productive in their lives. She was among the early writers to stress how time-limited groups placed special demands on the worker to clarify purposes and goals within the limitations of time; and, to focus on content, preparation and structure to make best use of time.

The purposeful use of time in social work was perhaps most apparent in the "functional" approach identified with the University of Pennsylvania, which, as Ruth Smalley (1971) pointed out, early advocated the need for workers to affirm and exploit each and every passing moment so as to attain its fullest unique value. In the course of living, with all things temporal, there can be generated a "readiness for what now looms as a new beginning of other ventures, with their promise, hope, and opportunity for using what has been experienced" (p. 1203).

Group workers in this tradition emphasized the need to help group members assess and use the validity of time—especially as it was played out in the group process—as a critical dynamic in the helping process. Time was an essential component in the social group worker's repertoire of skills. As Helen Phillips (1973) pointed out, workers needed to be able to use time in exploiting present reality, in exploiting time phases for group development, in utilizing structures, and in helping members deal with the trauma of endings and new beginnings. Throughout, it was the worker's sense of "rhythm" of the group process that was important (Ryder, 1976).

Time variables are also recognized as important in current group work models. The responsibility of the worker to monitor time as a resource, for example, is amplified in mediating approaches. Time is most often identified with task-centered and crises intervention orientations applied in short-term treatment. Time-limits, in the task-centered approaches, are used to establish the length and frequency of service. Time is decisive from the start as the work of the group is focussed on achieving the task—which is the ultimate criterion of success. The crises intervention model similarly stresses the time factor as it focuses on helping people regain a more balanced equilibrium at a particularly vulnerable period in their lives.

Although time-limited groups are not entirely new to social group workers, only recently have we begun to identify certain common features in group work with time-limited groups that are shared by workers with differing orientations working in diverse settings. As the reader will note, these common features are reflected throughout the articles presented here: the specification of achievable goals, utilization of time pressures, structured use of time, worker directedness, intensification of relationships, accelerated group processes and group development, etc.

Defining Time-Limited Groups

The concept of the time-limited group has varied meanings. In the first place, no specified amount of time has been established to distinguish between time-limited and other kind of groups. In fact, the basic definition of a group has been stated to be "two or more persons in interaction around a commonality of time *however brief*" (Casper 1983). And so duration is not the key determinant of what makes for a group. While time-limited groups are distinguished from time-unlimited groups that go on indefinitely, the distinction—strictly speaking—does not hold, for all groups eventually come to an end and are therefore time-limited.

Time-limited groups often are taken to mean "short-term" or "brief treatment" groups. However, it is not always clear what is meant by the terms "short" or "brief" inasmuch as the meaning and significance of time differs. Some time-limited groups may not have been planned to be limited as such but turn out to be prematurely terminated or aborted unexpectedly. These need to be differentiated from those that are consciously planned to terminate at a pre-determined point in time. Some time-limited groups consciously use time as a factor in the group process and again, these should be differentiated from those that are time-limited only in the sense that they are scheduled to fit into some pre-determined time period where there is no deliberate effort to use time as a factor in the group process. In general, then, a conventional time-limited group might be defined as a group that is formed with some sense of purpose and time length specified, and contracted in advance.

The concept of "on-going" groups usually conveys the notion of a time-unlimited group where members may come and go, but where the group continues on "indefinitely." However, any given member's participation may be taken to be "time-limited" and experienced as time limited. But again, unless there is a deliberate use of time in the process, the experience may be viewed as time-unlimited.

The single session group would appear to be a classic example of the short-term, time-limited group to the extent that the time limitation is consciously used in the process. It is at least conceivable that a single session group, such as a "one-shot" group meeting, may not connote the same sense of immediacy a single session time-limited group experience might. Single session groups therefore set unique kinds of limits. The constraints of time are circumscribed by different reasons, but the time constraint is still there. The single-session group has its own beginning, climax and end, which can be used to accomplish goals that would be facilitated where time is used as a concrete resource or tool. That which applies to short-term groups also applies to the single session group. The major difference being in the higher degree of sensitivity, energy, and risk taking in scaling down expected outcomes, the quickened pace with which the group is encouraged to move through group development, and the deeper intensity of engagement in the group.

Groups with changing memberships create a special case of the single session group. Inasmuch as the memberships can vary from session to session, the operating time line is realistically one session at a time each with its own beginning, climax and ending. Outcomes do not depend on continuous memberships. Instead, open member- ship groups function as a series of single session groups that begin and end whenever someone enters or leaves the group which changes groups composition and interactive potential.

Meanings of Time

Although basic to our existence, time has been ambiguously de- fined and takes on varying biological, physical and psychological meanings. At least two conceptions of time have prevailed over the years: the first, identified with the Aristotelian tradition, stresses time as an objective variable that, although continuously in motion, is absolute and quantifiable; the second, traced from St. Augustine through Einstein's theory of relativity to contemporary phenome- nologists, hold that time is relative and multifaceted and is internal- ly experienced as "subjective." Similarly, writers distinguished between "categorical" and "existential" time, the former being equated with "real" time sometimes called "adult" time while the latter is equated with "child" time which is "endless and eternal" (Mann and Goldman, 1982). Researchers have generally found that the crucial variable that differentiates subjective estimates of tem- poral intervals are not related to age so much as it is to variables such as activity levels, socioeconomic status, intelligence, education and other external factors (Hendricks and Hendricks, p. 36). Clear- ly, language and cultural orientations affect time perspectives. And as it is recognized that the process of socialization is the primary factor that contributes to one's temporal perspectives.

Although we might personally experience time in different ways, our experiences are not isolated and independent from others. Clear- ly we function in a society and culture which consists of systems of references that more or less uniformly influence our temporal ties and relationships. The picture is further complicated by the fact that we use a variety of time perspectives which are applicable to differ- ent arenas in our life space—such as the physical, psychological and social.

The subjective significance of time would appear to be a critical variable in working with time-limited groups. And yet, the current literature continues in the tradition that takes time to be an absolute quantifiable variable—something divorced from the consciousness of the observer or participant. Few writers, for example, address the need for workers to get a sense of the "subjective" time of the various group members or of their own time perspective, for that matter. Models of time-limited group work tend to ignore variables regarding members' personalized meanings of time, perceptions regarding duration, frequency and speed of time, subjective reactions to time under varying conditions, and so on. The failure to take subjective time perspectives into account would also throw into question the efficacy of certain time-limited principles that simply assumes that members are prepared to respond to time limits, are prepared to scale down goals, accept boundaries and make other uses of time.

To the degree that a group is greater than the sum of its parts, it is not unusual to expect that given the presence of personalized subjective times, in interaction where there is the sharing of values, the emergence of a group culture, norms, contagion, etc. a common subjective group time could evolve. It is conceivable that members who share similar experiences are more likely to share such a common "time" clock, although, of course, it should not be taken for granted that a common frame of reference will have similar influences on all members. For doubtless, there will be variations depending upon the degree to which members are implicated in the group, the roles and statuses that are occupied, identification with sub-groups, marginality and other group variables.

And finally, time-limited group experiences cannot be viewed as isolated experiences divorced from the network of group experiences of which it is a part. Group processes are by no means limited within the small group.

Framework

The following framework is offered as a simple device for arranging one's views about working with time-limited groups. From the multitude of definitions, perspectives and hypotheses, three major premises emerge. The first comes from an external world view which holds that time limits can be accepted as real boundaries that can be used positively. The second reflects a changing view of group interactions which emphasizes the concurrent ongoing processes. The third premise stems from the worker's mission as a helper which uses high intensity activities to make better use of the group within limited time.

The crucial factor in the first premise is the worker's willingness to consciously use known-in-advance time limits as an independent variable, an unchangeable "given" in the experience of the particular group. By divorcing time from the group, a specified amount of time in a time-limited group can become the boundary (within which there can be endless freedom) as well as the potential catalyst (unchanging) for effecting change.

The second premise focuses on enhancing services to time-limited groups by exploiting the concurrent existence of "stages of group development" whether, for example, they are labeled "forming/storming/norming/performing" Tuchman, 1965); "initial/convening/formation/conflict/maintenance/termination" (Henry, 1981); or the well-known "preaffiliation/power and control/intimacy/differentiation/termination" (Garland, Jones and Kolodny, 1965). It is valuable to note that there are indicators of all stages of these dynamics (unique to working with groups compared to working one-to-one) visible to some degree at all times in every group (Casper, 1983, Hartford, 1972) (see Figure 1). Therefore, the omnipresence and constant evolution of all stages of group development imply that a worker can view these phenomena as potential resources to be

Figure 1

Concurrent Evolution of Stages of Group Development
Using the Garland, Jones, Kolodny (1973) Components

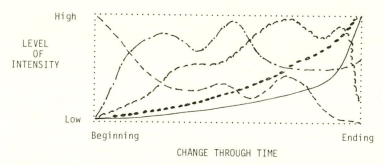

Coding:

Preaffiliation indicators ___ ___ ___ ___   Intimacy indicators ∿∿∿∿∿∿∿∿∿
Power and control indicators _.._.._..__   Differentiation Indicators ●●●●●○
                                                Termination indicators _____

- Casper (1983)

used as tools, contexts, vehicles, or targets—all of which offer special leverage for social work practice with time-limited groups.

In addition, "each time span (such as an eight-session group) has within it smaller spans (single sessions), each with its own beginning, climax and ending, and also episodes within sessions (such as a new decision, an agenda item, a surprise visit) with similar evolutions. Specific indicators may be almost imperceptible, but 'fine tuning' of the worker's observation skills, coupled with his/her knowledge and judgment, can make them available on behalf of the group" (Casper, 1983).

The third premise, one that highlights the worker's stake in the helping service, infers that both limited time and group interactive potential call for alert, complex, and perhaps risky efforts on the part of the worker. Higher intensity is seen as the coping strategy for relatively limited or reduced time with a group if substantial goals are to be reached. Given this rationale for high intensity, we can hypothesize support for the view that "group" is more valuable when viewed as a "practice resource"—defined here as a flexible supply that has adaptable characteristics, rather than as "practice 'method'"—which tends to be "habitual" and seen as an "established" approach (Gero, 1984).

This higher-intensity rationale, in turn, further enhances the utilization of the strengths inherent in groups. Furthermore, intensive efforts with time-limited groups are better focussed on preventive energies and supportive activities, since these are benefits the group members can transfer more readily to other parts of their lives.

For the worker, these higher performance expectations translate into greater personal resources and greater flexibility in their applications. As with the sophisticated camera which can change to cope with almost any external situation, workers are more effective when they can muster varied skills to cope flexibly with the desires and needs of the time-limited group.

These skills, when appropriate to group purpose and motivation, may take such forms as (1) role taking (trying out in the group some social behaviors that have personal meaning in everyday situations; (2) rehearsal—choosing and trying out projected future actions and decisions; or (3) helpful performance feedback—including descriptive, specific, timely communication that is solicited and willingly accepted by the receiver (see Casper, 1983).

A most powerful tool for transforming time limits into useable group assets is "the sensitive increase in the intensity of the group experiences, provided this is based on the worker's knowledge, skill, and values of caring and concern for human dignity'' (Casper, 1983).

Practices reflect a range of prototypes which implicitly, if not explicitly, claim to increase the potentials for success. The picture is complicated by our inability to capture the essence of the true meaning of success which is reflected in our lack of agreed upon definitions of success criteria in our work. But even if we were able to agree on the benefits of time-limited group experiences, it would not mean that we could always tell why some are helpful while others are not. Nor would it be clear that the time-limited approaches were superior to those that did not make similar use of time. In spite of everything we have learned over the years about the way group experiences impact people's lives, the interpersonal dynamics are extremely complex and elude our efforts to isolate and control group properties, processes, events and happenings that will ensure reliable and predictable outcomes.

These two themes—the need to examine the definitional and conceptual problems inherent in any assessment of time-limited group experiences; and the need to develop a frame of reference that will help us trace and relate significant group variables to preferred outcomes—represent important items on our agenda for the future.

If there is any central thesis, it is that our ability to assess the efficacy of time-limited group experiences will continue to be limited as long as we lack agreement about criteria linking such group experiences to results that are both predictable and reliable.

Overview of Contributions

The contributors to this edition give various reasons why time-limited group work may be the treatment of choice. There seems to be general agreement that such groups are economical or cost-effective at least to the degree that they require less expenditures of staff resources. The frequent use of time-limited groups to ''establish boundaries,'' may echo the need for structure that can take advantage of the ''sense of immediacy'' and other subtle pressures inherent in shorter group experiences. To the extent that the group experience makes conscious use of time limitations, it provides ''boundaries'' which have clearly perceivable influences on group members. Explicit reference to time pressure seems to encourage more structured use of time, it highlights the need to streamline and specify goals that are achievable, and implies greater reliance on workers to help make good use of time in structured ways. Still another theme that emerges is the recognition that short-term group experience bears the advantage of reducing dependency in groups.

The rationale for time-limited groups is often argued on pragmatic grounds. Time-limited groups may be offered to patients, for example, who are only available for certain periods of time—while sitting in a waiting room or at certain intervals while being oriented, examined, treated, discharged, or whatever. In such cases, the time factor fits naturally enough into a larger overall treatment program wherever members are processed.

The goals, on the whole, tend to be more specific and limited. Time limits are used to establish boundaries which facilitate structures that are more suitable to achieving specific individual and group goals. Interestingly enough, the nature of the problems addressed, as spelled out, are not really that different from what might be expected in time-unlimited groups. Both time-limited and time-unlimited groups are used to respond to a variety of needs whether focussed on the complex needs of children of divorced parents, depressions experienced by college students, clients coping with interpersonal stress, loneliness, isolation, disability, role transitions, etc.

In practice, time-limited groups do not appear to be limited to any particular orientation—existential, behavioral, analytic; nor does there appear to be any clear identification with any one "model" or approach. Methods and techniques typically identified with social behavior, crisis intervention, task-centered or traditional social group programming—are extensively used. Group formats differ considerably. Some are co-led while others are led by single workers. Generally, workers play more active roles in structuring content and influencing group processes. Most pay particular attention to group development and the need to make good use of "accelerated" processes. This applies to single-session as well as open-ended models.

In all of the groups presented here, the length of time is strictly determined. Many of the approaches work in extremely short time dimensions of the single session groups. In the more usual pattern, groups meet from six to twelve sessions. Still others use time-limitations in groups that are in reality "open ended" memberships. From the worker's standpoint, preference for time-limited approaches is apparent although relatively little is done to compare the outcomes of time-limited to time-unlimited groups. What can better

be done in ten as against twelve sessions, for example, is not established nor is it likely that precise differences will be made until we
are ready to make more systematic comparisons controlling a host
of varibles influencing the process.

Practice Notes

A sample of vignettes that describe actual practice experiences
are presented here in the form of "practice notes" to reaffirm the
need to keep our practice with time-limited groups grounded in the
real world.

These practice notes provide brief illustrations of practice which
consciously use time-limited group experiences in meeting the needs
of differing populations in diverse settings. Goals focus on social
growth and development, treatment, prevention, self-actualization,
problem-solving, staff training and development, etc. Group members include children, adolescents, adults, who are seen individually
and as members of families as well as groups. Some of the methods
address personal anxieties, stress, depression, loneliness, low-self
esteem; some deal with interpersonal relationships, parent-child
conflicts and problems; others are specifically focussed on helping
physically and mentally ill people, alcoholics, disabled and handi-
capped populations; still others focus on problem-solving, education, self-actualizing potentials, and so on. The settings include
hospitals, clinics, child-guidance centers, child welfare programs,
community-based supportive services, public schools, specialized
educational programs including professional training and instruc-
tional programs. While all confine services to relatively short time
periods (usually less than ten sessions) interventions and orientations
differ as alternative ways of dealing with group structures, development, programming, etc., are highlighted.

Future Directions

Where do we go from here? Contributors to this special edition
describe a variety of practices and procedures and offer many in-
sights into what can be done to make for successful time-limited
group experiences. The work that has been done to date is promis-
ing. Yet, there are many questions to be answered in setting future
directions.

Questions persist in at least three broad areas: (1) impact of agency practices on time-limited groups; (2) client characteristics and reactions; and (3) worker preparedness and involvement. Some of the kinds of questions to be addressed would include the following:

Agency Practices: What are the "appropriate" goals or expectations of time-limited groups? Are there significant differences in regard to agency settings, functions, resources? What is the relation of time-limited group successes to the availability of resources, service decisions, third-party payment influences, etc.? How significant are agency's "back-up" supportive services in the process?

Client Responses: Do clients feel better or less served in time-limited groups? Are there "appropriate" clients for such group services? What population factors are important—personality dynamics, age/sex, ethnic variables?

Worker Involvement: Which factors affect worker's performance and readiness to work with time-limited groups? What new skills, knowledge training is required? How does worker attitude affect the process? Can specific worker intervention be identified with successful time-limited group experiences? What is the meaning of time to the worker? How do workers react to partial successes? How do they react to subtle agency pressure to render services within time constraints, etc.?

Although not easily answered, such questions need to be addressed if we are to demonstrate the efficacy of the time-limited group experience in the growing repertoire of activities essential to the practice of contemporary social group work.

Albert S. Alissi
Max Casper

REFERENCES

Casper, M. (1983). The Short-term Group: A Special Case in Social Work. In N. Goroff (Ed.), *Reaping From the Field—From Practice to Principle. Proceedings of Social Group Work Three—1981*, Vol. 2. Hebron, Connecticut: Practitioner's Press.

Garland, J. A.; Jones, H. E.; and Kolodny, R. L. (1973). A Model for Stages of Development in Social Work Groups, in *Explorations in Group Work*, Saul Bernstein (Ed.). Boston: Charles River.

Gero, A. (1984). *A Group Resource Model*. Paper presented at the Annual Program Meeting of the Council on Social Work Education, Detroit, Michigan.

Hartford, M. E. (1972). *Groups in Social Work*. New York: Columbia University Press.

Hendricks, C. D. and Hendricks, J. (1976). Concepts of Time and Temporal Construction Among the Aged, with Implications for Research. In F. Gulbrium (Ed.), *Time, Roles, and Self in Old Age*. New York: Human Sciences Press.

Henry, S. (1981). *Group Skills in Social Work: A Four-Dimensional Approach*. Itasca, Illinois: F.E. Peacock.

Mann, J. and Goldman, R. (1982). *A Casebook in Time-Limited Psychotherapy*. New York: McGraw-Hill Book Company.

Moyle, H. B. (1946). Some Psychiatric Comments on Group Work, *The Group* 8(2), 1–4.

Phillips, H. (1957). *Essentials of Social Group Work Skill*. New York: Association Press.

Ryder, E. L. (1976). The Functional Approach in *Theories of Social Work with Groups*, Robert W. Roberts and Helen Northen (Eds.). New York: Columbia University Press.

Shoemaker, L. (1960). Use of Group Work Skills with Short-Term Group, *Social Work with Groups*, New York: National Association of Social Workers.

Smalley, R. (1971). Social Casework: The Functional Approach, *Encyclopedia of Social Work*, New York: National Association of Social Workers, pp. 1195–1206.

Tuckman, B. W. (1965). "Developmental Sequences in Small Groups," *Psychological Bulletin*, Vol. 63.

Wilson, G. and Ryland, G. (1949). *Social Group Work Practice*. Hebron, Connecticut: Practitioner's Press—Reprint 1981.

Time-Limited Treatment Groups for Children

Steven R. Rose

ABSTRACT. Children with psychosocial problems relating to school, health, and mental health difficulties have been treated in time-limited groups. The present article explicates the process of small group treatment with children using the time-limited approach. The objectives, establishment, planning, and composition of groups as well as the leadership, activities, termination, and evaluation of these groups is presented.

In recent years, the helping professions have been subjected to a variety of forces that have influenced clinical practice. Social work and the other helping professions have been faced with the challenge of demonstrating that their services are genuinely helpful to clients (Pardes & Pincus, 1981). Environmental and professional trends have contributed to the development of time-limited clinical social work practice (Wells, 1982). It was discovered that the realities of clinical practice are such that much unplanned time-limited treatment occurs (Beck & Jones, 1973; Garfield, 1980; Parad & Parad, 1968; Verny, 1970).

Corresponding to trends that contributed to the development of time-limited treatment, social and professional forces led to the growth of small group interventions. The purpose of the present article is to describe the use of time-limited groups in the treatment of children. A review of the professional literature is included and a conceptualization of time-limited group treatment of children is developed. Social problems experienced by children that are amenable to time-limited treatment in groups are discussed. Numerous aspects of clinical group practice, including the setting of objectives, the es-

Steven R. Rose, MSW, PhD, is Assistant Professor, Social Work Program, University of Vermont, 451 Waterman Building, Burlington, Vermont 05405.

tablishment of groups, planning the format, joining of children, member composition, leadership, process, ending of meetings, and evaluation are presented.

Characteristics of Time-Limited Group Treatment of Children

Time-limited group treatment with children is a mode of intervention that has numerous salient characteristics (see Wells, 1982). The focus of the approach is usually circumscribed. Practitioners deal with a set of problems that are frequently managed within a relatively brief time frame. The approach is often useful for children who have little access to traditional, extended-time interventions. Those with limited resources of time and finances are generally able to use a time-limited approach.

Positive pressures can be experienced by practitioners to identify problems, develop objectives, and work productively. Treatment is usually explicit, deliberate, and planned. The social workers attempt to attain a limited number of goals for the child's benefit. The general objectives of time-limited group treatment are to achieve a positive change in the current life of the child, relieve stress, and reduce demoralization.

Use is frequently made of either personal or behavior change methods that are derived from crisis intervention or social learning theories, respectively. As in crisis intervention the focus of time-limited clinical practice is often a pressing or urgent difficulty presented by the child. The intervention process includes goal-setting, intervention, and termination.

The group aspects of a time-limited strategy offer several advantages in working with children. Small treatment groups are generally more attractive to children than interactions between one child client and one adult practitioner (Rose, 1972). Groups can be efficient and effective means of helping more than one child at a time.

Small groups can be settings in which children simulate the responses and reactions of the real world. Children frequently have the opportunity to practice patterns of thinking, witness emotional responses, try out new social behaviors, and receive feedback from their peers. Social learning readily takes place in the protected environment of the group setting. The presence of other children with related difficulties affords a measure of social reality. Activities practiced in the protected environment of the small group can be employed in the members' social world.

Treated Social Problems of Children

Time-limited treatment groups have wide applicability for social work interventions with children. First, these types of groups have been useful for children of divorce (Titkin & Cobb, 1983). Such children experience emotional responses consisting of a sense of powerlessness, depression, distress, sadness, joylessness, regression, and aggressive acting-out (Titkin & Cobb, 1983).

A second type of difficulty addressed in time-limited children's groups is social competence (Rose, 1982). Interventions have been developed to help children learn to make and keep friends (Lewis & Weinstein, 1978) and resolve interpersonal conflict (Edleson, 1981).

A third set of clinical problems that can be resolved in time-limited children's treatment groups are health-related. Work has been done with children who have emotional and behavioral disorders (McCarnes & Smith, 1979). Also, families with children born with spina bifida have been helped (Bergofsky, Forgash, & Glassel, 1979).

Finally, children who were involved in delinquency have been treated in children's groups that are time-limited (Ross & Bilson, 1981). Such groups can be useful in assisting children who have been either the victims or the perpetrators of sexual assault.

Group Objectives

Time-limited treatment groups for children have established objectives. These include the broadening of children's understanding of divorce and the normalization of the experience of parental divorce (Titkin & Cobb, 1983). Other objectives for children have been the recognition and healthy expression of feelings (Titkin & Cobb, 1983) and the ability to give and accept physical expressions of warmth (Ross & Bilson, 1981).

Skills are frequently the focus of time-limited groups for children. Development of abilities has been sought in the following areas: friendship skills (Lewis & Weinstein, 1978), interpersonal skills for conflict resolution (Edleson, 1981), social skills (McCarnes & Smith, 1979; Rose, 1982) and cognitive skills (Rose, 1982).

An additional objective has been for children to explore new ways of handling conflict, and the development of cooperation, sharing, and trust (Lewis & Weinstein, 1978). Children have been taught

self-control, to develop creative play with one another, and to enhance their relationships with adults (Ross & Bilson, 1981).

Group objectives also include increasing children's awareness of
how their actions influence peer responses as well as improving
children's self-esteem (Lewis & Weinstein, 1978). The treatment of
emotional and behavioral disorders can be an objective as well (Mc-
Carnes & Smith, 1979).

Establishment of Groups

The objectives of time-limited children's groups are usually established in conjunction with an assessment of needs and matching
these needs with resources (Ross & Bilson, 1981). In some cases,
need assessment is done on a formal basis. For instance, a survey
was done of "children on social workers' case loads who were at
risk of . . . being taken away from home by the courts and having
to live in a residential institution" (Ross & Bilson, 1981, p. 16). In
another case, a medical diagnosis of spina bifida in children prompted
the sending of a letter to the homes of clinic families (Bergofsky et
al., 1979). In a third case, school social workers and teachers observed children in upper elementary school experiencing frequent
unresolved conflicts (Edleson, 1981).

In some instances, social work practitioners treated children experiencing difficulties that could be met through time-limited groups.
Clinicians at a child guidance clinic discovered children without
friends (Lewis & Weinstein, 1978). Practitioners at a community
mental health center worked with children who were experiencing
emotional and behavioral disorders (McCarnes & Smith, 1979).

When children's difficulties stem from parental social problems,
services provided for adults can expand to those offered to children.
Eleven years following the establishment of social services for sepa-
rating and divorcing parents, a children's program was offered. It
was based on the assumptions that the adjustment of children following divorce is influenced by the parents and that latency-age children in general are influenced by their parents (Titkin & Cobb,
1983).

Planning the Group Format

After assessing the need for children's services, social agencies
can develop group programs to increase the effectiveness of their
services (Bergofsky et al., 1979). Time-limited group work as an

approach is generally chosen for several reasons (Lewis & Weinstein, 1978; Ross & Bilson, 1981). The approach is often beneficial for children with related problems and similar assessed needs for intervention. For children who know each other outside of the group, the special features of a time-limited approach can be utilized. The group provides a support system for the children. Members "support and encourage each other between sessions and after the end of the group" (Ross & Bilson, 1981, p. 17). A buddy system can be used. Furthermore, when a group is composed of children who are referred for having similar problematic behaviors, such as delinquency, the setting is usually employed to develop a new set of norms. Finally, the time-limited nature of the group experience permits a focus on a limited number of explicit and achievable goals, such as the development of friendship skills (Lewis & Weinstein, 1978).

Social agencies employ time-limited approaches to the group treatment of children as an alternative to providing long-term services such as activity group therapy (Lewis & Weinstein, 1978). Time-limited approaches to clinical group practice with children usually involve a relatively brief amount of time spent in direct interaction. The number of sessions ranges from 6 to as many as 20 with 12 being a more usual upper limit (Edleson, 1981; Ross & Bilson, 1981). Groups meet once or twice a week. Weekly sessions allow time for children to try out new behaviors developed in group sessions. With younger children more frequent meetings allow greater continuity of person, place, and events. The length of group sessions varies between 45 and 90 minutes. Shorter sessions are often preferable for younger children who have briefer attention spans. Time-limited groups can be designed to produce rapid personal or behavior change that tends to occur when meetings are held frequently over a brief period of time. Intensity of intervention appears to lead to faster progress (Lewis & Weinstein, 1978).

The speed of progress for children may be linked to securing the involvement of parents (Ross & Bilson, 1981). In some cases of children's work, time-limited groups for parents are the focus of intervention (see Bergofsky et al., 1979). In time-limited group treatment of children, a range of parental involvement occurs. In some instances parents merely give their permission for their child to be treated (Edleson, 1981). In other cases, full parenting programs are offered in conjunction with children's groups (Titkin & Cobb, 1983). A determining aspect of parental involvement appears to be the nature of the presenting problem. When the child's difficulties are directly related to problems experienced by the parents, as in divorce, a program for parents is sometimes offered, whereas when they are indirectly related to parental problems, as in children's adjustment problems in school, an adult program is rarely offered.

In addition to planning the degree of participation and involvement of parents, the practitioners consider the level of structure to be used in the group. In general, time-limited groups for children are highly structured (McCarnes & Smith, 1979). They tend to be designed to make efficient use of meetings. The group format reflects the daily social lives of children with their everyday problems (Lewis & Weinstein, 1978).

Practitioners employing the time-limited group approach make conscious use of the physical environment for helping children. Groups have been offered in settings such as a non-profit counseling agency (Titkin & Cobb, 1983), a medical clinic (Bergofsky et al., 1979), the group room of a youth guidance center equipped with a one-way mirror and a rug serving as a base for group ritual (Lewis & Weinstein, 1978), the statutory public social welfare department in England (Ross & Bilson, 1981), the downtown unit of a community mental health center (McCarnes & Smith, 1979), and classrooms in elementary schools (Edleson, 1981; Rose, 1982). The diversity of these environments reflects the wide applicability of a time-limited approach with children. Each setting has been the focus of social service provision for children with particular needs.

Joining of Children

Planning group services is usually a precursor to their implementation. A process of intake involving assessment of children is frequently employed. In the time-limited group treatment of children the intake process can be integrally related to the type of services provided by the social agency. For instance, when a child receives a medical diagnosis of spina bifida the social work department of a health clinic can offer social services to the family (Bergofsky et al., 1979). In school settings, teachers can refer children with social skill difficulties to social workers (Edleson, 1981; Rose, 1982).

Social workers also play a more direct role in bringing children to time-limited treatment groups. Referral by therapists within a clinic to a group has been shown to be effective (Lewis & Weinstein, 1978). In mental health agencies children are often placed in time-limited groups as part of their treatment (McCarnes & Smith, 1979).

In public social welfare settings, the need for time-limited clinical group services has been recognized. A combination of referrals from within the welfare agency and from other agencies, including police and youth services, has been used effectively (Ross & Bilson, 1981).

In time-limited group treatment with children the assessment process is usually rapid. It includes at least one interview with the child. In some instances parents and children are interviewed. Questionnaires, checklists, and family drawings made by the child are often used (Titkin & Cobb, 1983). If contraindications exist to placing the child in a group, or if the child does not meet the criteria specified for group membership, he or she can be screened out and referred either for individual services or to another type of group.

Group Composition

For those children who are appropriate for time-limited intervention, frequently it is the task of the group leaders to compose the group. Generally, the treatment groups consist of girls and boys (Lewis & Weinstein, 1978; McCarnes & Smith, 1979). Mixed gender composition accurately reflects the real social world of children. It allows children to learn to interact constructively with others regardless of gender.

Groups are usually formed of children within one or two chronological years of one another. Intellectual and emotional development are sometimes considered in combination with actual age and grade level (McCarnes & Smith, 1979).

The treatment groups consist of a balance which allows the characteristics of children to complement each other. At a youth guidance center a time-limited group was composed of girls and boys who were aggressive and withdrawn, or overprotective and overprotected (Lewis & Weinstein, 1978).

The range of socioeconomic status of group members is often wide in settings where medical disability determines eligibility for services (Bergofsky et al., 1979). The range has tended to be more narrow in certain school systems (Rose, 1982) and in public child welfare settings (Ross & Bilson, 1981).

Group size tends to be between four and seven children although larger groups can be composed (McCarnes & Smith, 1979). In schools, classrooms can be subdivided into small groups for effective practice (Rose, 1982).

Group Leadership

Although group meetings can be led by one practitioner they are usually conducted by two practitioners (Bergofsky et al., 1979; Bilson, 1981; Edleson, 1981; Lewis & Weinstein, 1978; McCarnes & Smith, 1979; Rose, 1982; Ross & Bilson, 1981; Titkin & Cobb, 1983). The advantages of a pair of leaders conducting group sessions include having extra support and perception available to the adults and greater opportunities for the children to see adults working together in a trustful and communicative manner (Lewis & Weinstein, 1978). In larger groups, two leaders help keep the group on-task and productive (Rose, 1982). The group leaders can be either staff or interns (Bergofsky et al., 1979). Occasionally, the group leaders use a consultant or supervisor to indirectly assist with the group process (Bergofsky et al., 1979; Ross & Bilson, 1981).

Group Process

After composing the group, the practitioners direct their activities according to the phase of group development. The beginning sessions often serve multiple purposes. The leaders develop a forum for mutual sharing, establish group structure, promote trust, and help the group develop cohesion and commitment (Titkin & Cobb, 1983). The children engage in readiness activities that include playing games and roles, observing others, making suggestions, and giving feedback during group meetings, as well as completing assignments between meetings (Edleson, 1981).

The middle sessions are usually devoted to problem-solving, discussion, role playing, puppetry, communication skills, board game playing, and drawing (Titkin & Cobb, 1983). Skill training is frequently conducted through the use of assignment cards, a point system, problem-solving, brainstorming, roleplaying, modeling, coaching, feedback, and summarizing (Edleson, 1981). Growth games, discussion, drama, video, creative play, and journals are often useful in the operation of the group (Ross & Bilson, 1981).

Group Ending

The termination phase of the group process involves structured generalization (Edleson, 1981; Titkin & Cobb, 1983). It consists of at least one session.

In time-limited clinical practice with children the length of the treatment group is usually announced at the beginning (Ross & Bilson, 1981). When the group ends the members are likely to feel varied emotions, including sadness, and can be encouraged by the leaders to express their feelings about the ending of the group. The members' responses may reflect feelings of loss they have experienced in their young lives. Some children demonstrate relapse behaviors. However, dependency problems tend to be less apparent in time-limited groups than in other types of children's groups (Ross & Bilson, 1981).

The leaders assess the group members' readiness for termination. The children maintain their skills, integrate concepts, and apply the knowledge they have gained. Through game-playing a process of review occurs. Selected leadership activities can be transferred to the members. Teachers, parents, and siblings are sometimes included in meetings. After the group ends, booster sessions and periodic newsletters can be useful means of maintaining the progress that children have attained in treatment (Edleson, 1981).

Evaluation of Group

Following the termination of the time-limited children's treatment group, an evaluation of its effectiveness can be completed. Typically, this consists of assessing the process and outcome of the group. Usually objective data and subjective impressions are combined in an overall assessment. In-group and out-of-group changes of children are usually noted. Reports from peers, parents, social workers, and teachers are frequently used. Evaluation designs tend to be before and after quasi-experimental, or pre-post experimental in nature.

Positive results of time-limited children's groups have been obtained. Ross and Bilson (1981) observed much case by case clinical improvement at a public welfare agency. Fewer problems were reported outside the group. Within the group setting, children could concentrate, there was no fighting, warmth was expressed, and fears were verbalized. At a community mental health center McCarnes and Smith (1979) noted significant improvement on parts of a parent's questionnaire and of a teacher's questionnaire as well as on a global rating by the group leader.

Lewis and Weinstein (1978) found observable changes in children at a youth guidance center. They saw an improvement in group participation. Aggressive children were helped through the treatment group.

Studies in school settings also support the efficacy of the time-limited approach. Edleson (1981) reported that peers and teachers observed greater improvement by children in skill training programs when compared to an activity group program. Rose (1982) indicated that teachers noted improvements in the social behaviors of children in social skills groups. Greater achievement motivation and less aggression, anxiety, isolation, and overall disability were reported on teacher's checklists.

At a counseling agency Titkin and Cobb (1983) noted decreases in tantrums, anger outbursts, withdrawal from peers, bedwetting, and excessive clinging. Positive changes were reported in school performance, mood fluctuations, sibling relationships, problem-solving skills, identification of feelings, and the communication of feelings to parents. Within the group, attendance and enthusiasm remained high and disruption decreased.

Conclusions

The time-limited approach to group treatment of children has considerable utility. Stemming from the need for more efficient use of practitioner resources, the approach has proved valuable in helping children with diverse psychosocial difficulties. Establishing time-limited treatment groups has become more feasible in recent years as social agencies have adopted a brief intervention model. The overall objectives of time-limited clinical groups have been to promote the social functioning of children and to minimize the deleterious effects of educational, health, and mental health difficulties. Multiple factors exist in the planning, composing, leading, and ending of these children's treatment groups. Evidence exists to support their effectiveness.

Time-limited treatment groups provide social support to children with similar, rapidly assessed needs for intervention. Small groups tend to be composed of girls and boys similar in age, intellectual development, and emotional development. Pairs of leaders help children through the use of a range of activities appropriate to the levels of group and individual development. The ending of time-limited clinical groups usually involves a consolidation of treatment gains that have been made by the children. Evaluations of treatment groups often include a formal and positive assessment of outcome.

REFERENCES

Beck, D. F., & Jones, M. A. (1973). *Progress on family problems.* New York: Family Service Association of America.

Bergofsky, R. E., Forgash, C. S., & Glassel, A. F. (1979). Establishing therapeutic groups with the families of spina bifida children in a hospital setting. *Social Work with Groups, 2,* 45-54.

Edleson, J. E. (1981). Teaching children to resolve conflict: A group approach. *Social Work, 26,* 488-493.

Garfield, S. L. (1980). *Psychotherapy: An eclectic view.* New York: Wiley.

Lewis, K., & Weinstein, L. (1978). Friendship skills: Intense short-term intervention with latency-age children. *Social Work with Groups, 1,* 279-286.

McCarnes, K., & Smith, L. L. (1979). Evaluating a children's group treatment program. *Social Work with Groups, 2,* 343-354.

Parad, H. J., & Parad, L. J. (1968). A study of crisis-oriented planned short-term treatment, Parts I and II. *Social Casework, 49,* 346-355 & 418-426.

Pardes, H., & Pincus, H. A. (1981). Brief therapy in the context of national mental health issues. In S. H. Budman (Ed.), *Forms of brief therapy* (pp. 7-22). New York: Guilford.

Rose, S. D. (1972). *Treating children in groups.* San Francisco: Jossey-Bass.

Rose, S. R. (1982). Promoting social competence in children: A classroom approach to social and cognitive skill training. *Child and Youth Services, 5,* 43-59.

Ross, S., & Bilson, A. (1981). The sunshine group: An example of social work intervention through the use of a group. *Social Work with Groups, 4,* 15-28.

Titkin, E. A., & Cobb, C. (1983). Treating post-divorce adjustment in latency age children: A focused group paradigm. *Social Work with Groups, 6,* 53-66.

Verny, T. R. (1970). Analysis of attrition rates in a psychiatric outpatient clinic. *Psychiatric Quarterly, 44,* 37-48.

Wells, R. A. (1982). *Planned short-term treatment.* New York: Free Press.

Transition to Parenthood:
A Time-Limited Mutual Aid Group
to Facilitate a Major Role Change

Nancy Boyd Webb

ABSTRACT. Time limits, task assignments and mutual aid under-
pinnings form the basis for this six-session model of group work,
specifically adapted to meet the needs of parents-to-be. Grounded
philosophically in the developmental life model of social work practice, this time-limited mutual aid group approach incorporates elements from Schwartz' reciprocal (mutual aid) model, crisis, and
task-centered approaches. The article stresses the preventive implications of group support and psychological preparation for couples
in the critical period of their transition to first-time parenthood.

Time is the silent language that speaks of potentiality and limits, of creativity and death, of change and permanence. (Carel
Germaine, 1976)

Couples expecting their first baby are keenly aware of time and
its passage. Their attention and thoughts are riveted upon the specified due date which will transform them irrevocably from a couple
into a family. Some are very nervous about the future birth itself,
and about its subsequent major responsibilities. Others center their
dreams and expectations on the pleasure of the anticipated child,
without considering the major upheaval a dependent baby will create
in their lives.

Despite the wide range of possible individual reactions, becoming
a parent is a profound role transition for all. It constitutes a crisis for
many, and is a milestone for which most couples are very poorly
prepared. Jack Bradt (1980) states that "becoming a parent is a major nodal event in the family life cycle. Nodal events, like all chal-

Nancy Boyd Webb, DSW, is Assistant Professor, Fordham University Graduate School
of Social Service, New York, NY 10023.

lenges, have the potential to stimulate growth and strengthen the family system or to stimulate dysfunction.''

This article proposes the use of a time-limited (six session) group to assist couples who are anticipating the birth of their first child. The proposed group is grounded philosophically in the developmental life model of social work practice (Germaine and Gitterman, 1980) which recommends offering help during life's critical transition points. This group work approach was created specifically to assist parents-to-be. Our time-limited mutual aid model incorporates elements from the following three group work approaches:

1. The Reciprocal (Mutual Aid) Model (Schwartz, 1961)
2. The Crisis Group (Strickler and Allgeyer, 1967; Parad, Selby and Quinlan, 1976)
3. The Task-Centered Approach (Garvin, Reid and Epstein, 1976)

After a brief review of the need for parenthood preparation, we will argue the appropriateness of time-limited mutual aid groups for couples undergoing this major role transition. The special role of the leader will be specified, and we will propose a specific structure for the group sessions, which includes one separate meeting for the group of husbands alone and one for the group of wives, in addition to four sessions with the couples together.

Need for Parenthood Preparation

> Although the transition to parenthood may not be as much of a trauma or crisis as it was thought to be a few years ago (Le-Masters, 1957; Hobbs, 1976), it is still a tremendous shift for the couple, and one they are often unprepared to make (Rossi, 1968). . . While couples have the period of courtship to prepare for marriage, *there is virtually no direct preparatory experience for having a baby.* (McGoldrick, 1980, emphasis mine)

Even family life education workshops seem to overlook this significant milestone and opportunity for prevention. A 1982–83 publication list of The Family Service Association of America, for example, fails to present any programs specifically earmarked for the couple awaiting the birth of their first child. In contrast to the plethora of childbirth preparation courses typically available in most communities, programs addressed to the mental health and shifting emotional strains of expectant parents are virtually non-existent. While guidance for the birth experience itself is certainly important, these courses simply do not provide attention to the marital relationship and to the *psychological* preparation for parenthood which the significance of this major life event merits.

Studies by the Feldmans (1977) on the effect of parenthood on the marriage relationship of 850 middle-class couples from an industrial large city in the northeast showed that those who were parents had a significantly lower level of marital satisfaction. The role strain of parenthood was particularly hard on couples whose relationship was judged very close before parenthood. The child came between them and threatened their closeness. Many had not explored their individual attitudes about child rearing which often proved to be highly divergent, and another source of conflict. The Feldmans comment that "since parenthood is such a demanding and important task, it probably should not be entrusted to amateurs. Those who become parents should have some training for the task" (Feldman, H. and Feldman, M., 1977). They recommend the use of neighborhood groups, classes and discussion groups as social supports to facilitate adjustment to the parenting role.

The Feldman report confirms the author's practice experience in a mental health setting working with preschool children and their parents. History-taking often reveals that problems began or came to a head with the birth of the first baby.

> Mario was not the same man after we had Carmen, said one client. He became agitated, moody, incomprehensible, angry. He could not understand that although I still loved him, things had changed. Now Carmen was here and she needed not only me, but him also. She was so fragile. He was convinced that Carmen had replaced him. I think that's the reason he left.

This example, while extreme, conveys both the stressful impact of the baby's birth and the lack of preparation for it. Even when desired and eagerly anticipated, the change in family structure from a dyad to a triad inevitably causes an upset of the couple relationship and, therefore, creates a crisis state.

A review by Naomi Golan (1981) of several studies by family sociologists since the mid-1950s tried to determine whether or not young couples considered their adjustment to the recent birth of their first child as a crisis situation. Early research (LeMasters, 1957; Dyer, 1963) indicated that this did constitute a crisis for many; more recent studies (Hobbs, 1965, 1976), however, found different results, with most couples reporting only "moderate or low levels of crisis" associated with the birth of their first baby. These latter studies prompted Golan to view the entry into parenthood as a transitional stage, rather than a crisis.

Regardless of terminology, becoming a parent clearly constitutes a new and different status with added duties and expectations for performance. Holmes and Rahe's (1967) scale of life adjustment includes pregnancy as a significant life stress which often is associated with other important stresses such as a change in residence, a change in work status, and increased financial strain. Reuben Hill (1958) maintains that the addition or loss of any individual member in a family causes a necessary realignment of roles, and hence qualifies as a crisis.

It appears that the verdict is still uncertain regarding whether or not the transition to parenthood is a crisis, and if it is, how extensive a crisis it represents. Perhaps differing definitions of crisis account for some of this disagreement, since most lay people consider a crisis to be a catastrophe, whereas trained crisis workers usually subscribe to Rapaport's 1962 definition of crisis as an upset of a steady state.

This broader view leads directly to the possibility of providing anticipatory guidance as a preventive measure to help people plan ahead for predictable future stressful situations. Janis' research on medical patients who were awaiting surgery (Janis, 1958) suggests the value of "anticipatory fear," since it often leads to appropriate information-seeking behavior. Doering and Entwisle (1975) applied Janis' theory to women undergoing childbirth and found that mothers who had sought knowledge beforehand required less medication during labor and delivery. It is the position of this article that preparation for psychological changes implicit in the transition to parenthood will result in parents who are more knowledgeable, more comfortable and more effective in their new roles than had they not engaged in this preparation.

The Model

The author's interest in crisis intervention and prevention, which was the focus of an earlier paper on Crisis Consultation (Webb, 1981), prompted the design of a time-limited mutual aid transition to parenthood group, intended to provide both support and information. The group offers expectant parents the opportunity to discuss their anxieties and expectations about parenthood with peers, who thus become a source of mutual aid. Members are encouraged to enlarge their repertoire of coping skills by learning from one another and by seeking information from other sources when this is appropriate. The leader is a facilitator, who keeps the group focused and helps stimulate discussion. Intended for the population-at-large, the ideal meeting place is a "Y," church or any community facility where a room with comfortable chairs and privacy can be ensured.

Announcements about the group may be advertized in local newspapers, posted on appropriate bulletin boards in the community, and flyers can be left in the waiting rooms of cooperating obstetricians. Information on the announcement includes the time and place of group meetings and procedure for registering.

Since this is a formed group, with no pre-group screening, it is important to give sufficient information in the announcement to enable prospective participants to understand the purpose and goal of the group.

This is a model of the announcement which can be printed on a flyer, with specific information regarding meeting place and registration on the bottom half of the notice:

The Transition to Parenthood: A Discussion Group for First-Time Parents

A discussion group for mothers and fathers-to-be. Focus will be on preparation for the anticipated role transition from "couple-status" to "family-status" identity.

This group is based on the conviction that recognition and discussion of natural concerns about parenthood promotes a climate of mutual support which will strengthen the couple's interaction and effectiveness as future parents.

Subjects for group discussion include the following:

— maintaining meaningful communication
— jealousy
— changing sexual needs and responses
— sharing responsibilities
— dealing with future grandparents
— enhancing intimacy and the marital bond

This is not a therapy group, and couples who are experiencing severe marital problems are not encouraged to register.

Enrollment will be limited to seven couples to facilitate maximum participation of all members.

The group will meet on six consecutive Thursday (or other) evenings from 8:00–9:30 P.M. The first two meetings will consist of all couples together; the third meeting is for wives alone, and the fifth is for husbands alone.

The First Session

As with any beginning group, introductions are important, as is an initial statement about the purpose and goal of the group ("to help you help each other with your concerns, expectations, hopes and fears about becoming parents"). The leader will take an active part in making introductions, stating the purpose, facilitating the discussion, and helping the group articulate common worries as a basis for establishing the contract. The fact that the couples have registered, having seen the announcement, indicates general interest and agreement about the over-all thrust of the group. However, it is still the worker's responsibility to verbalize the purpose of the group, and to help individual members clarify more specifically how the group can assist them with their individual concerns.

The worker will indicate that the meeting plan offers the opportunity for husbands and wives to meet separately from each other (one session for each) in order to focus more specifically on gender-related issues about parenthood (i.e., what it means to a man to become a *father*, and to a woman becoming a *mother*).

Thus it should be clear to all by the end of the first meeting, and the leader may wish to summarize, that the group will deal with issues which concern *all parents-to-be* as they anticipate undertaking the parenting role, in addition to *individual* worries and concerns, and also *gender-related* topics. These different foci constitute the work of the group during the six-session structure.

The introductions in the first session should include an invitation to each member to say something about how it feels *right now* to be anticipating the birth of a child. In all likelihood this will result in various references to feeling about becoming a parent (mother or father). Since a major focus in this first session is on recognition of the significance of this status and role change, we have devised several "exercises" to facilitate this awareness. Leaders may choose to use these or not, depending on personal preference and the mood and climate of the particular group. The exercises are as follows:

1. *"Free Association"*

— Leader hands out paper and pencils.
— Asks members to fold paper in half.
— Leader asks group members to "free associate," then jot down all words or phrases they connect to the word "parent." A second association, immediately following on the other half of the folded paper is to the word "spouse."
— Comparison of the lists provides an interesting lead-in to discussion of the distinctive role differences between the two statuses.

2. *"Expectation and Reality"*

— This is a guided fantasy exercise.
— Leader asks couples to recall their expectations three months prior to their marriage, and to then compare that memory with the reality of their subsequent experience.
— The purpose of the exercise is to expose the romantic and often unrealistic expectations about marriage and parenthood which may make the reality appear jarring by comparison.

The author believes that use of these free association and fantasy exercises will stimulate discussion and move the group into a greater level of intimacy than typical of initial group sessions.

At the end of the first session, members will be asked to think about and prepare a list of at least five ways in which their lives will change after the baby's birth. They will be expected to share this with the group during the second meeting, and to identify the two changes which they believe will be the hardest for them. It will be the work of the group in the second session to help members plan a coping strategy to deal with their primary concerns.

The Second Session

The reporting back to the group of the individual lists of concerns forms the focus of this session. The procedure of "going around," while somewhat artificial, nonetheless ensures that everyone participates and receives the benefit of the group's concentrated attention, for a brief period of time. It also serves the purpose of affirming the capacity of each member to offer support to the others, and, inevitably realizing that one's own innermost worries are often identical to the concerns of others. This facilitates the bonding process in the group.

The worker's task during this session is to point out the common ground and to help the group help each other. Some workers may use a chalkboard, or large writing pad, on which to record the major concerns of each member. This permits later over-all comparison and identification of similar concerns among members.

Since the next meeting will be with the wives only, a carry-over *task assignment* for both husbands and wives will be to find and talk to someone who has had a baby in the last year. Women will talk to new mothers and men to new fathers. They should ask and take notes about the most difficult and most pleasurable experiences of the new parents during the first three months *after* the baby's birth. This will serve as the focus of the segregated discussions during the third and fifth weeks of the group meetings.

Third and Fifth Sessions

These meetings are special because they provide prospective parents a place to talk about concerns that are specifically gender-related. Although some practitioners may believe that it is contra-indicated to break up the group in this manner, the position of the author is that the potential gains outweigh the disadvantages. Each spouse is, of course, free to share with the partner at his or her discretion, aspects of discussion which seem pertinent to their relationship. The leader will have the responsibility to relate issues back to the entire group in a general way, insofar as it seems appropriate to do so.

The goals of both these sessions is to look ahead to the actual experience of parenthood and also to have a safe place to talk about their special concerns about the pregnancy itself. The worker should state this dual purpose at the beginning of the sessions so that the members understand that both future and present are fair game for discussion. Since each member has been instructed to speak with a new parent about the joys and frustrations of the first three months of parenthood, this is a logical beginning point for the discussion.

After a reasonable amount of time, the leader can shift the discussion from the future to the present by asking how members are actually experiencing the pregnancy period.

The psychiatric literature (Anthony, 1970) is an important resource for the worker in preparation for the separate sessions with the prospective mothers and prospective fathers. The concensus is that the concerns of each sex about parenthood are somewhat different, and may be difficult to share with the spouse.

The following letter printed in a newspaper advice column might be used as a discussion stimulus for the men's group:

> My wife and I have planned our baby, but now that the time is approaching when it's really going to happen, I'm a nervous wreck. I know this is the time that I'm supposed to play the role of the strong, supportive male, but I can't recall ever having felt less like that. I'm filled with anxiety about whether or not I'll be able to face my new responsibilities and I honestly just wish I could shut myself up in a quiet room alone, and forget the whole thing. Obviously, I can't, but now I realize why some men drink more when their wives are pregnant. The pressures are enough to drive me to drink. Is this normal?

The unique worries of pregnant women often focus on changes in their body configuration, much of which gets transformed into worry about weight gain. Fears of loss of physical attractiveness are very common. There will be relief in sharing these concerns in the women's group. The worker may wish to use a quote such as the following, to lead into discussion of these issues:

> I've felt so dragging. I'm very uncomfortable and just wish it were over with. I feel like I'm tripping over my belly and I can't support the weight anymore. It's hard to stand up, and it's hard to lie down. . . . I'm never tremendously happy and sometimes I get depressed. (Grossman, et al., 1980)

The worker should ask each separate group to decide the content of the report back to the spouses regarding the nature of their discussions. The worker's responsibility is to bridge the separate and larger group sessions by sharing selected content from the separate meetings.

Fourth Session

The group is now past its mid-point and the worker needs to acknowledge this, and again ask each member to indicate if and how any of their views on their transition to parenthood are changing as a result of the group discussions and their own evolving perspectives. This stock-taking and re-assessment is important for the leader to encourage. An additional responsibility of the leader is to recognize that there will be one more session (number six) with the entire group together. The leader may suggest that each member come to that last session prepared to state one new coping technique he or she has learned as a result of being in the group. This is presented as a task assignment for the final meeting.

Sixth Session

This session will begin with a review of these individually learned coping strategies, some of which undoubtedly will overlap with those of others. Again, a chalkboard or large note pad will be helpful. The leader who kept notes during the second session about the individual concerns of each member can use these to help the group identify increased understanding and individual progress in appropriate preparation for the parental role.

As the group prepares to say goodbye to one another and to the leader, some inevitably will wish to remain in contact with one another; most will want to know about the birth of each other's baby. The group may exchange addresses. The real termination of the preparation for parenthood is, of course, the birth itself.

The leader should highlight and praise the mutual help which the group gave and received, indicating that this helping process can continue informally, without the structure of planned meetings.

Worker Activity

As has been clear in the previous description of the worker's role, the author views this as an active, facilitating, mediating function appropriate for this time-limited mutual aid group.

The worker is quite active and directive, keeping the group working on the original goal and purpose: to help them help each other with the transition to parenthood. In a mutual-aid group the worker's chief contribution is to set the helping process in motion and to promote its continuation.

The worker's movements must reflect the movements of others, as he acts to help others act. His moves are directed toward specific purposes, limited in scope and time, and touching only those within his immediate reach. (Schwartz, 1961; 185)

Linkages with Other Group Work Models

The time-limited mutual aid model presented here has its roots in three distinct group work models: Schwartz' reciprocal (mutual aid) model, Strickler and Allgeyer's crisis group format, and more recent adaptations of this (Parad, Selby and Quinlan, 1976), and Garvin, Reid and Epstein's task-centered approach, which is an outgrowth of Reid and Epstein's task-centered casework (1972). Elements from each of these models combine in this specially created blended approach.

A common emphasis in all three models is the planned use of time which is particularly apropos here considering the obviously time-limited state of pregnancy itself. Crisis and task-centered approaches deliberately use time as a motivating force in promoting change, whereas the reciprocal (mutual aid) model stresses the important role of the worker in monitoring the time phases of the group (beginning, middle and end). The six-session format also represents time boundaries, and is a time frame typical for crisis groups.

The role of the worker in this blended model balances an active, directive stance (typical of crisis and task-oriented workers), with a willingness to validate and encourage the contribution of each individual member to one another (a strong emphasis in the mutual aid model). Utilization of the group to help individual members solve or work on their problems is a vital component of all three approaches.

Expectations for change are implicit in all helping efforts. Schwartz refers to "the demand for work" (Schwartz, 1976), Parad, Selby and Quinlan (1976) view the development of new coping means as an important focus for crisis groups, and Garvin, Reid and Epstein (1976) discuss use of the group process to help members formulate and attain tasks.

Conclusion

Unique in neither its structure nor method of work, the time-limited mutual aid model presented here does claim originality in its identification of important unmet need, and in its development of a group work approach explicitly designed to fit that need. It is ironic that the currently popular modish emphasis on the life cycle and its passages has not produced programs or services specifically designed to help couples make the transition into parenthood.

The time-limited mutual aid model of group work presented here fills a service gap and offers exciting opportunities for primary prevention in its focus on fostering realistic attitudes of parents-to-be about their children-to-be.

REFERENCES

Anthony, E.J. & Benedek, T. (1970). *Parenthood: Its psychology and psychopathology.* Boston: Little, Brown and Company.

Bradt, J.O. (1980). The family with young children. In E.A. Carter and M. McGoldrick (Eds.), *The family life cycle* (pp. 121–146). New York: Gardner Press.

Doering, S.G. & Entwisle, D.R. (1975). Preparation during pregnancy and ability to cope with labor and delivery. *American Journal of Orthopsychiatry, 45*: 825–837.

Dyer, E. (1963). Parenthood as a crisis: A re-study. *Marriage and Family Living, 25*:2, 196–201.

Feldman, H. & Feldman, M. (1977). Effect of parenthood at three points in marriage. Presentation and mimeo paper. American Orthopsychiatric Association.

Garvin, C.D., Reid, W., & Epstein, L. (1976). A task-centered approach. In Robert W. Roberts and Helen Northen (Eds.), *Theories of social work with groups* (pp. 238–267). New York: Columbia University Press.

Germain, C. (1976). Time: An ecological variable in social work practice. *Social Casework, 57*:7, 419–426.

Germain, C. B. and Gitterman, A. (1980). *The life model of social work practice.* New York: Columbia University Press.

Golan, N. (1981). *Passing Through Transitions* (pp. 80–98). New York: The Free Press.

Grossman, F.K., Eichler, L.S., & Winickoff, S.A. (1980). *Pregnancy, birth and parenthood.* San Francisco: Jossey-Bass.

Hill, R., (1958). Generic features of families under stress. *Social Casework, 39*:2, 139–150.

Hobbs, D.F. (1965). Parenthood as a crisis: A third study. *Journal of Marriage and the Family, 27*:3, 367–372.

Hobbs, D.F., & Cole, S.P. (1976). Transition to parenthood: A decade replication. *Journal of Marriage and the Family, 38*:4, 723–731.

Holmes, T., & Rahe, R. (1967). The Social readjustment rating scale. *Journal of Psychosomatic Research, 11*, 213–218.

Janis, I.L. (1958). *Psychological stress.* New York: Wiley.

LeMasters, E.E. (1957). Parenthood as Crisis. *Marriage and Family Living, 19*:4, 352–355.

McGoldrick, M. (1980). The joining of families through marriage: The new couple. In Elizabeth A. Carter and Monica McGoldrick (Eds.), *The Family Life Cycle* (pp. 93–119). New York: Gardner Press.

Parad, H.J., Selby, L. and Quinlan, J. (1976). Crisis intervention with families and groups. In Robert W. Roberts and Helen Northen (Eds.), *Theories of social work with groups* (pp. 304–330). New York: Columbia University Press.

Rapoport, L. (1962). The state of crisis: Some theoretical considerations. *Social Service Review, 36*:2, 211–217.

Reid, W.J. & Epstein, L. (1972). *Task-centered casework.* New York: Columbia University Press.

Rossi, A.A. (1968). Transition to parenthood. *Journal of Marriage and the Family, 30*:1, 26–39.

Schwartz, W. (1961). The social worker in the group. *The social welfare forum* (pp. 146–171). New York: Columbia University Press.

Schwartz, W. (1971). On the use of groups in social work practice. In William Schwartz and Serapio R. Zalba (Eds.), *The practice of group work* (pp. 3–24). New York: Columbia University Press.

Strickler, M. & Allgeyer, J. (1967). The crisis group: A new application of crisis theory. *Social Work, 12*:7, 28–32.

Webb, N.B. (1981). Crisis consultation: Preventive implications. *Social Casework, 62*:8, 465–471.

The Neighborhood Group:
A Reminiscence Group
for the Disoriented Old

Lorrie Greenhouse Gardella

ABSTRACT. This reminiscence group helped disoriented old people find intimacy with others in the present time. Telling of loss, group members resolved grief by seeking meaning in their experience. Folktales allowed the group to reminisce even when memories failed. The group's time limited structure helped the worker empathize with old people's life tasks. But time limits were not useful to a group whose members had little awareness of calendar time.

You want to hear the story of my life? I tell you, everyday I tell myself the story of my life. I tell it to the walls of my room. This place is all right. They leave me alone. But it would be no trouble to me if you come and listen. (Mr. S., age unknown, The Jewish Home for the Aged)

When I was a social worker at The Jewish Home for the Aged, clients told me stories of their lives. Despite losses of mental and physical faculties, losses of memory or disorientation in space and time, clients tried to remember. They told stories of loss: losses of families, friends, homes, and losses of physical and mental faculties. They told of the loss of memory itself. The old in the nursing home not only remembered; they also tried to tell of their experience to others. Reminiscence was both a private and a social activity. Through self expression, expression of oneself in the past, the old patients affirmed self images and found intimacy with others, alleviated crises and worked toward integrity: "the ego's accrued assurance of its proclivity for order and meaning" (Erikson, 1963, p. 268).

Lorrie Greenhouse Gardella, JD, MSW, is Team Associate Director, West Haven Community House, West Haven, CT 06516.

I worked with clients, aged eighty to one hundred three years, who had been diagnosed as having some form of organic brain damage (e.g., Organic Brain Syndrome, Arteriosclerotic Senile Dementia). These diagnoses did not necessarily describe the condition of the brain itself. As Feil explains, "in old old age (over eighty years) the condition of the brain alone often bears little relation to the behavior of the living person. Behavior in old old age is a combination of physical, social, and emotional factors" (Feil, 1981, p. 7; Monsour and Robb, 1982, p. 412).

Diagnoses such as Organic Brain Syndrome described patterns of behavior: gradual losses of orientation in space and time, of recent memory, of the ability to think rationally, or of the ability to express emotions in socially acceptable ways. When under stress, whether physical or emotional, some clients withdrew from others, ignoring the present and "living in the past." When stress was alleviated, as in music therapy or in art therapy, clients felt less disoriented. Engaging in social activity, clients became interested in the present, regaining linguistic and social skills.

I was assigned to form a time limited group for clients with whom I worked for the purpose of improving the quality of life on the floor. Objectives of the Neighborhood Group, as we called it, were to provide a social environment where clients, however "confused," would feel that their lives in the present were worthwhile, and where clients who often withdrew into the past would find intimacy with others in the present time.

Not surprisingly, group members discovered one another in the process of exploring the past. Reminiscence became the natural language of a group whose members sought integrity as a life task. The time limited group became a group for making sense out of time.

This paper explores the value and functions of a time limited reminiscence group for the disoriented old. Further, it suggests that reminiscence groups as they are offered to mentally alert old people may be adapted to the needs of the disoriented old by sharing folk stories in addition to personal stories. For folk stories evoke stories of our own lives.

In the Neighborhood Group, reminiscence and the expression of reminiscence to others proved as valuable to disoriented clients as to those mentally acute old people who generally are invited to recreational "reminiscence groups" (see, for example, Ingersoll and Goodman, 1980, p. 308.) While telling or listening to each other's life stories, the disoriented old found a freedom of affect and a fluency with language which often was lost to them in day to day life at the Home. Attention spans grew and concentration deepened. Reminiscence gave old people a means to affirm their self image—I am who I was—. They showed each other not only frailty but also lives of achievements and strengths.

Discovering or rediscovering their own lifelong worth, clients became interested in each other. Reminiscence led to intimacy in the group and to friendships which extended beyond group sessions. In the once silent lounge, clients conversed.

"Well, it used to be a bunch of old strangers, here," one client observed.

The opportunity to tell about the past brought disoriented clients from the past to the present, for, in the present, they would be heard. As Feil writes:

> If (the disoriented old) cannot express feeling to someone in the present time, they will express feeling to people they recreate from the past. . . If no one listens, the feelings continue. If someone listens, the feelings are validated and often subside. (Feil, 1981, p. 19)

Reminiscence in the Neighborhood Group alleviated some of the loneliness of the disoriented old. The importance of such an activity lay partly in its power to transcend a client's life. In telling her story, a client, however isolated, could leave her story as a legacy in the minds of others (Butler, 1975, p. 418).

While the disoriented old reminisced as a recreational and social activity, they also used reminiscence to resolve crises past and present. In the process of telling and listening to each other's life stories, the Neighborhood Group found opportunities for what Butler calls "life review":

> the progressive return to consciousness of past experiences, in particular the resurgence of unresolved conflicts which can now be surveyed and reintegrated. (Butler, 1975, p. 412)

As the old review their lives, Butler adds, "they frequently experience grief. The death of others, often more than their own death, concerns them" (Butler, 1975, p. 412).

One crisis occurred in the Home when the husband of a beloved head nurse died unexpectedly. Clients grieved for the nurse's loss and for their own losses of family and friends. Suddenly, clients with chronic illnesses suffered particularly severe symptoms, and clients in relatively good health fell ill. During the next week, every client with whom I met told me of her own awakened grief for a spouse, a child, or a friend who had died long ago.

I offered this observation to the Neighborhood Group, a group whose members had outlived many—and sometimes all—significant others. Through reminiscence, clients in the group mourned publicly for the family and friends who had died.

Mrs. B. began the discussion by describing her last conversation with her husband:

"He was just going out to buy a newspaper. But he went out the door and he never came back. . . If only I knew then that he would never come back."

In listening to each other's story, clients felt newly aware of their feelings for past and present losses. They relived the experience of mourning and expressed anger, guilt, loneliness, and a sense of irremediable loss.

The intense feeling of grief allowed clients' egos to focus on objects lost in the past. The ego could identify with the lost object, freeing psychic energy for creative uses.

One creative use of psychic energy was narrative. For some, the expression of feeling alleviated grief. Reminiscence with others became an opportunity to make "reparation" and to lessen feelings of guilt. As Butler explains:

> Older people are constantly writing and rewriting the scenarios of their lives. Sometimes chased by the furies of guilt, they try to resurrect and come to terms with regretted actions of commission and ommission out of their past. (Butler, 1974, p. 417)

In narrative, the old found a "second chance."

The disoriented old tried to preserve tenuous memories of lost objects in words and to put their memories in order. Narrative helped ease clients' sense of loss. Psychic energies were directed to listening as well as telling, allowing clients to feel intimacy with one another. Listening for their story in the stories of others, group members felt less alone. Energies were directed then to learning, as clients shared their adaptive styles:

"Sometimes I cried but I went where no one would see me. That's what Mrs. D. (the head nurse) will do."

"It's not so bad to cry . . ."

As reminiscence continued, tension gradually ebbed. Clients talked about their lives as widows, about trying to make new friends:

"Sometimes Mrs. G. here and I would go to the corner for an ice cream. We lived in the same apartment. Do you remember, Mrs. G.? Those were good times, before we had to come here (to the Home)."

After trying to accept a past and a present death, members of the group "returned" to the Home in the present time.

The Neighborhood Group did not appeal to all clients, and the session described here did not help all participants resolve crises or find self affirmation through intimacy with others.

After Mr. B. expressed in the group his love for his deceased wife, he left the room.

"It is too much *tsorus* (trouble)," said Mr. B.

Like the widow who went away to cry, Mr. B. did not want to mourn in public. Having listened to reminiscence in the group, however, Mr. B. did want to share his memories and feelings to someone who would listen. After the group, he told me how he met and how he lost his wife. From then on, we met in the empty dining room in late afternoons, and Mr. B., cigar in hand, told me of his experience, present and past. Through an intimately felt relationship, Mr. B. reminisced, expressed emotions, and measured his accomplishments. In itself, the desire to leave a legacy or gift to a younger person motivated Mr. B. to put his memories in order. Mr. B., like members of the group, looked for meaning, in part, in order that I could benefit from his experience.

Mr. B., then, was not comfortable when he tried to reminisce with the group. After experiencing the group, however, he wanted to express his feelings to another. The group indirectly helped Mr. B. come out of his silent grief for losses of the past.

Mr. B. was typical of most clients in that he was a good judge of his own appropriateness for the Neighborhood Group. Luckily, I trusted the clients' judgement. For it would have been impossible for me to predict who among the disoriented old would be capable of intimate relationships with several people in the present time. In most recreational groups, including art and music therapy, clients related to one person, the worker, forming strong and trusting bonds with her, but not necessarily with each other. Thus behavior of clients in the Neighborhood Group differed markedly from their behavior in other structured and unstructured settings at the Home. The process of reminiscing in the group gave clients a rare opportunity to care for and to be cared for by one another.

Two qualifications for membership in the Neighborhood Group emerged: (1) the desire to participate, and (2) the ability, which could not have been predicted, to feel and express intimacy with others in a group. The following criteria would have been *irrelevant* if I had tried to predict which clients would enjoy sharing stories of their experience: (1) disorientation in space and time, (2) difficulties in expressing oneself in words (e.g., aphasia), (3) hearing impairment, (4) a preference to listen rather than to speak, (5) physical pain, (6) wandering behavior, (7) disparities in clients' physical or intellectual abilities.

A skillful worker can learn patience along with the aged. She can help clients with language impediments find the lost words and she can encourage clients to help each other. Using a microphone or sitting near hearing impaired clients, the worker can translate what others have said in a low clear voice. The worker can respect listening, for listening may be as active and interactive a form of participation as speaking. In some settings, the worker can arrange for clients who are in pain to leave the meeting at will, planning with nursing staff to have help with transportation as needed. The worker can reserve seats for those who "wander," affording them the opportunity to come and go (Monsour and Robb, 1982). The worker can invite to the group clients with a wide variety of abilities and disabilities, whether physical or mental. For one client's weakness will be complemented by another client's strength.

Having composed the group, the worker must find a balance. On the one hand, she tries to engage clients in the activity of reminiscence. On the other hand, she must respect the judgment of the disoriented old as to the nature and quality of their participation in the group.

Reminiscence in a group allows the disoriented old to use the ego defenses which have enabled them to survive for many years. And reminiscence in a group allows clients to let go of some defenses, trying new means for survival. When a disoriented old person has relied primarily upon the defense of denial, she may repress memories in order not to feel pain. In a reminiscence group, denial as a defense is challenged. Clients are invited not only to express their own memories, but also to listen to the memories of others. A client may see in the face of another the pain she has denied for years.

Respectful of the old person as survivor, the worker should respect the client's lifelong style of ego defense. The group offers the old person reminiscence as an opportunity to review the past. But the choice between keeping defenses or letting them go belongs to the client alone.

In order to keep the invitation open, I found it helpful to visit clients before meetings of the Neighborhood Group. I reassured clients before and during meetings that I would help them return "home" to their rooms when the meeting was over. Meetings were short, rarely exceeding thirty minutes in length. After meetings, I spent time with each group member, as I accompanied her "home" or to the clients' lounge, where reminiscing sometimes continued after meetings had closed.

The Neighborhood Group offered activities related to but other than reminiscence. Diversity helped stimulate interest. The nursing staff contributed speakers on such topics as physical changes in aging and intellectual changes in Organic Brain Syndrome. Clients engaged in lively dialogue with speakers. Here they, the old, were the acknowledged experts on old age.

While seminars stimulated thinking, the telling of folktales stimulated feeling. The loss of recent memory or of other intellectual abilities did not make it impossible for disoriented clients to reminisce. For the heart of reminiscence—and of the search for integrity—lay in the ability to feel, rather than in the ability to think in words. Reminiscence is the exploration of subjective truth.

In the beginning of group sessions, many in the group could not remember objective historical truth: dates of events, names of loved ones, the courses of important trips. The disoriented old needed a way to the past other than objective or intellectual memory. Folk stories, for some, became a way.

In listing themes in psychotherapy with older persons, Butler includes: new starts and second chances, death in disguise or disguised fear of death, awareness of the present rather than the future, grief and restitution, and guilt and atonement (Butler, 1975, p. 265).

The old must make peace with the past and lost chances if they are to reach integrity. They must find a meaning for loss or feel that loss is temporal. They must look for meaning in their experience. As Butler writes:

> After one has lived a life of meaning, death may lose much of its terror. For what we fear most is not really death but a meaningless and absurd life. (Butler, 1975, p. 420)

When memories are dim, life review becomes difficult for the disoriented old. Folktales told in the Neighborhood Group reminded clients of "the ordering ways of different times and different pursuits as expressed in the simple products and sayings of such times and pursuits" (Erikson, 1963, p. 268). Folktales, Erikson might have said, prepared a way to integrity.

The old in the Neighborhood Group identified with those who spoke of good and bad times in the past. Identifying with others allowed clients to work through their own unnamed losses. Similarly, the clients identified with protagonists in folktales, who went upon quests very similar to the quest for integrity. Folk characters travelled from initiation to separation to return; from severance to retirement to rebirth; or from subjection to release to compensation (Colum, 1944). Consider these journeys in relation to Butler's list of psychological themes of people in old age:

Journeys in Folktales	*Psychological Themes of the Aged*
Initiation/separation/return	New starts and second chances Fears of death; death disguised Grief and restitution
Severance/retirement/rebirth	New starts and second chances Fears of death; death disguised Awareness of present time Grief and restitution
Subjection/release/compensation	New starts and second chances Grief and restitution Guilt and atonement*

In addition to resembling psychological issues faced by the old, the paths of characters in folktales reflected some of the physical realities of aging. In folktales, losses which occurred on those difficult paths usually were restored. In this sense, folktales offered hope to those who identified with some heroic character.

Journeys in Folktales	*Losses in Aging*
Initiation/separation/return	Losses of significant others
Severance/retirement/rebirth	Losses of self (e.g. of physical and mental faculties)

---

*Fears of death might have applied here for Christian listeners.

Journeys in Folktales	*Losses in Aging*
Subjection/release/compensation	Losses of environment (e.g. of homes

According to Butler, the old perceive time as a series of phases, "a purposive sequence of changes in psychological development" (Butler, 1975, p. 411). For "only in old age can one experience a personal sense of the entire life cycle" (*Idem.*).

The protagonists in folktales completed their journeys. They echoed the clients' sense of time. Folktales offered a hope that one may complete the journey to ego integrity. To some disoriented old, folktales suggested the existence of a meaning in the subjective past and the possibility of putting one's past in order. After listening to folktales, members of the Neighborhood Group would tell of their experience as a story with a beginning, a passage, and a resolution. As the oldest client explained:

> A story is just a story, but this is a life story. It shows how the people suffered and how they came to a new part, where the suffering came to an end. (Mr. J., aged 103, The Jewish Home for the Aged)

Once I began a folktale by saying, "There lived a girl who had no mother."
"I don't have a mother," Mrs. S. said, in tears.
Other clients helped validate Mrs. S.' feelings. As Feil explains:

> When feelings are validated, the old old person shares the reasons for the feelings. A disoriented old old woman rocks back and forth yelling, "Ma, Ma, Ma." The worker validates the woman's need to call for her mother. The old old woman trusts the worker and now no longer yells for her mother. The disoriented old old has found safety with the worker in the present time. (Feil, 1981, p. 16)

Whether identifying with characters in folk stories or identifying with each other in life stories, members of the Neighborhood Group mourned their own losses. As we have seen, the awareness of feelings allowed clients to focus on lost objects, freeing energies for self expression. The disoriented old who felt isolated did not express themselves in the present time. But when disoriented clients felt intimacy with one another, they found a potential to affirm self worth. In caring listeners, clients found the motivation for putting memories in order and finding their meaning. As one client listened to another, she eased her own loneliness, and she prepared herself for new reminders and new awareness of loss.

The Neighborhood Group met for four months, until its members talked with each other outside the group, reminiscing from day to day. We learned in the group that as our memories fade, we may find integrity in intimacy. And we may find intimacy as we share with each other the stories of our lives.

REFERENCES

Bettelheim, B. (1976). *The Uses of Enchantment: The Meaning and Importance of Fairy Tales.* New York: Alfred A. Knopf.
Burnside, I. M. (1978). *Working with the Elderly, Group Processes and Techniques.*
Butler, R. N. (1975). *Why Survive? Being Old in America.* New York: Harper and Row.
Colum, P. (1944). Preface, *The Complete Grimm's Fairy Tales.* New York: Pantheon Press.
Erikson, E. (1963). *Childhood and Society* (Second Ed.). New York: W.W. Norton & Co., Inc.
Feil, N. (1981). *The Feil Method: Validation/Fantasy Therapy.* Cleveland: Edward Feil Productions.
Freud, A. (1966). *The Ego and the Mechanisms of Defense* (Revised Ed.). New York: International Universities Press, Inc.
Golan, N. (1978). *Treatment in Crisis Situations.* New York: The Free Press.
Ingersoll, B. & Goodman, L. (1980). History comes alive: facilitating reminiscence in a group of institutionalized elderly. *Journal of Gerontological Social Work, 2* (4), Summer, 305–321.
Koch, K. (1978). *I Never Told Anybody: Teaching Poetry Writing in a Nursing Home.* New York: Vintage Books.
Monsour, N. and Robb, S. (1982). Wandering behavior in old age: A psychosocial study. *Social Work, 27* (5), September, 411–417.
Weiss, R. (1973). *Loneliness: The Experience of Emotional and Social Isolation.* Cambridge, MA: The MIT Press.

When Time Counts:
Poetry and Music
in Short-Term Group Treatment

Nicholas Mazza
Barbara D. Price

ABSTRACT. Poetry, music and time used as therapeutic agents in short-term (seven sessions) group treatment are especially helpful in working with depressed college students. They provide a means to reduce dependency and establish boundaries compatible with agency limitations. Specific poetic techniques include (a) sharing a preexisting poem or song and inviting reactions; (b) construction of a group of collaborative poems. Further guidelines and suggestions are delineated. A case example of a group for moderately depressed university students is provided. Particular attention is given to the use of time, poetry and music to motivate and activate clients. The group developmental stages within a brief time frame are also examined. A discussion of strengths, limitations as well as practice and research implications conclude the report.

University students who utilize campus counseling centers often come with a presenting problem that includes depression. While this initial assessment may not indicate clinical depression, it can be viewed as a forewarner of more severe stress. Students may also have ambivalent feelings about seeking treatment, perhaps because of negative preconceived notions about counseling centers. It is important to intervene early to prevent more serious distress and to provide an early positive experience that can help engage clients in treatment. Time, therefore, may be a critical factor in both preventive and engagement capacities. Also, since the university counseling center often has time restraints, it usually offers some form of brief treatment rather than long-term therapy.

Nicholas Mazza, PhD, is at the Florida State University School of Social Work. Barbara D. Price, MSW, is at the Florida State University Student Counseling Center, Tallahassee, Florida 32306.

Because of the above factors, a short-term group treatment model was developed using poetry and pop music as ancillary techniques. This use of poetry and music in group treatment provides a non-threatening vehicle to help clients express feelings and thereby become engaged in treatment. By talking about a poem or song, one is beginning to share thoughts and feelings, thus reducing defenses. Time-limited group treatment itself can be a viable modality in working with depressed college students, because it provides a means to reduce dependency and establish boundaries compatible with agency limitations (i.e., realistic demands for service). The added use of poetry and/or music in this short-term group treatment can be helpful because it provides a necessary focus through which clients have an opportunity to deal with time in the present rather than in the past. Poetry can be utilized to elicit here and now reactions while extending both backward and forward in time (i.e., clients may relate past experiences promoting universality and share current feelings promoting self-disclosure). Dynamic connections between past and present can also be developed.

Overview

The use of poetry in group therapy has been noted in a number of descriptive reports (e.g., Bressler, 1983; Buck & Kramer, 1974; Lerner, 1982; Lessner, 1974). The use of popular music as an adjunctive therapeutic technique with adolescents and college populations has also been described (Boyum, 1978; Mazza, 1979, 1981; Santiago, 1969). While the empirical base for the use of music in therapy is substantial, for poetry it is just beginning to evolve (e.g., Davis, 1978; Edgar & Hazley, 1969; Mazza, 1981; Ross, 1977; Williams, 1978).

Buck and Kramer (1974) discuss the use of poetry as a means of facilitating group process. These authors also observed a cumulative effect wherein group members learned the procedures of using poetry in therapy and developed a sensitivity to group functioning. Lauer and Goldfield (1970) earlier noted this phenomena with respect to the role of creative writing in group therapy. Lessner (1974) noted that poetry acted as a catalyst in group counseling with college students. Mazza and Prescott (1981) describe the use of poetry and music with a couples group in a university counseling center. It proved helpful in breaking resistance and facilitating group process in a time-limited modality.

This report will review the specific techniques for using poetry and/or pop music in short-term group treatment. These techniques include (1) sharing a pre-existing poem or song, and (2) the construction of group poems. The group as a case example will be analyzed with respect to specific group developmental stages noted by Garland, Jones, and Kolodny (1965): Pre-affiliation, Power and Control, Intimacy, Differentiation, and Separation. A discussion of the advantages and disadvantages as well as practice and research implications will conclude this report.

The group consisted of six members (2 males, 4 females) with an age range of 18 to 36. All of the members were undergraduate students. Most of the members had previously enjoyed reading some form of literature and/or listening to music. The seven-week format was decided with a consideration of the academic calendar and time limits of the counseling center. Within the time frame of both the semester and length of group treatment, students would be facing deadlines, making decisions and completing tasks. Time could therefore be used as a treatment variable consistent with other student responsibilities. Each session lasted 1½ hours. The group was co-led by one male and one female social worker.

Model and Techniques

Poetry and/or pop music were used within a group treatment model that combined the selection of pre-existing poems/songs and the development of collaborative (group) poems (Mazza, 1981). The use of pre-existing poems (e.g., Stephen Crane's "If I Should Cast Off This Tattered Coat") was primarily based on the isoprinciple of selecting a poem that is close in mood to that of client (Leedy, 1969). This principle was extended to include group mood and particular themes that evolved. A cassette tape was used for the music technique. Copies of the lyrics and/or poems were provided to the group members.

The collaborative poem is generally used toward the end of each session. This involves the creation of a group poem with each member having the opportunity to contribute lines. The group poem is initiated by the group leader(s) asking for a predominant theme or feeling in the group session. The poems are later typed and copies are distributed to group members at the beginning of the subsequent session. This use of the collaborative poem toward the end of each session provided the opportunity to recount how the time was spent and to bring closure to the session. By distributing copies of the group's collaborative poem to members in the subsequent session, a time link is established. Members can choose to discuss the poem and/or move on to other areas. This model of poetry therapy is incorporated within a generic social group work treatment framework.

Case Example

First Session

This initial group session included introductory issues (e.g., review of time designated for group), definition of group goals, format and a general exploration of member concerns. The commonality of depression was acknowledged by group members through David Ignatow's poem "Brooding" which includes the lines, "The sadness of our lives. / We will never be good enough to each other, / to our parents and friends." Members were cautious in speaking, with minimal self-disclosures. The use of a pre-existing poem was helpful in providing some early structure and allowing members to talk about feelings in a nonthreatening manner. In this first session, the poem was helpful in establishing an atmosphere that promoted member participation (i.e., discuss and/or create a poem). This maximized the use of time available while dealing with personally meaningful issues that may have been of concern for a long time. Of particular importance was the attention given by members to the line "never be good enough." Time was viewed as hopeless with individuals being helpless in dealing with family relationships, academic failure and psychosexual issues. By beginning to identify and define their feelings, group members could perceive time in a more helpful (e.g., "I don't have to decide today" or "I reserve the right to change my mind later") and productive (e.g., we completed a poem today) manner. The collaborative poem would also prove helpful in subsequent sessions to signify the end of each session.

The group collaborative poem entitled "depression" included the following lines:

> . . . inside a sinkhole
> dark, grasping
> restless, listless, tired

don't want to do anything
. . . feel FAT and ugly
Why would anybody like me?

This poem reflected a collection of individualized feelings associated with depression. It is consistent with early group development in which members can maintain distance on the one hand, while becoming involved with other members in the commonality of depression.

Second Session

Power and control issues emerged during this session. One member (male) arrived late and maintained a posture of silence and noninvolvement. This nonverbal communication served to set the member apart while drawing attention from others to involve him in group discussion. At approximately the midway point in the session, one of the group leaders introduced Dave Loggins' song "So You Couldn't Get to Me" to the group. This song was consistent with both the theme (isolation) and mood (depression, frustration) of the group. The timing of the use of the song was geared to tap into the group process and facilitate forward movement. Also the melody of this song evoked a rather slow and relaxed pace that helped to reduce tension and allowed the group (above male member in particular) to express their feelings. The song includes the lines, "I wish I was an island and you could not swim / I wish I was a room that you could not get in." The silent member identified with the feelings expressed in the song. He began to share some difficult times he had experienced with a woman. Some members joined in supporting him while one member intellectualized and voiced negative feelings toward males. The song evoked personal reactions by most of the members. Group members were asked by one of the leaders: "If you had an island, who would you invite onto it?" A group member was able to establish some independence and provided an important issue of personal space by responding that she wouldn't invite anyone and that the question for her pertains to whom she would leave her island for in order to visit. This member was able to lessen her dependency on others while establishing the boundaries of the island.

The collaborative poem was entitled "Anger." It reveals an attempt to begin an examination of depression; however, there is little cohesion with contrasting lines (e.g., "Throwing stones at the moon/Energy not directed well. . ."). The collaborative poem was particularly helpful in this session in activating the silent and most visibly depressed member. He was asked to write down the lines for the group. This involved getting out of his chair and recording lines on a flip chart. The activity appeared to mobilize this member's energy and to heighten his affect as he became more verbal and participated in the creation of the poem.

Third Session

In reviewing the collaborative poem from the previous week, issues pertaining to the expenditure of time and energy were discussed. Particularly, some members were discontent about a disproportionate amount of time spent on some individuals. Quiet members were able to voice their needs and concerns by initially responding to the collaborative poem. Subsequently member and leader responsibilities were clarified with energy re-directed. Jim Croce's song "I Got a Name" provided some impetus and validation for the above expression. The melody of this song helped accelerate the pace of the session. Issues of identity, family and interpersonal relationships, and career options were brought up in the session.

The collaborative poem entitled "Relief" demonstrates the therapeutic value of the session. It also suggests the early development of trust in the group and subsequent challenges.

> ### Relief
> is voicing
> what you've been afraid to say.
> taking a weight
> off my back
> and feeling more free
> looking
> at the feelings that are ok
> are there any feelings
> that are not ok?
> sometimes
> I just don't know my feelings
> and that's ok too.

In effect, the last lines of the poem validated the confusion and struggle while the group continued to develop.

Fourth Session

This session involved more risk taking as more meaningful personal experiences were shared (e.g., difficulties in dealing with former spouse, parental pressures to attend college, feelings of inadequacy, etc.). Stephen Crane's poem "If I Should Cast Off This Tattered Coat" was used to help deal with the anxiety involved with risk taking and the unknown. The poem was helpful in dealing with the risk of expressing self in group. One member had been talking about her "writer's block" in completing a term paper. This was later used to connect to a "group block" in which it was difficult to express self. Issues of risk and trust were of central concern. The group responded to the image of the tattered coat, noting for some it was a secure coat. For others, they were ready to "go free into the mighty sky." Discussion included how some individuals were trying to "hold back the clock" to avoid possible rejection or failure. Mention was also made by the leaders of the group calendar (i.e., amount of weeks left in the group) and how time would be used to deal with the above issues. Essentially time was both a lever and point of discussion for the group.

The collaborative poem began this week without a title. It included the following lines:

> Conflicts with each other
>   delving into each other's feelings
>   wondering
>   mental blocks
>   Misunderstandings
>   having to explain
> Striving to understand each other
>   Different values
> Trying to be open-minded
>   trying to listen
> and be heard . . . maybe
> Accepted and accepting
>   Cloudy reasoning -
>   struggling with the cloud
>   With each other

Upon completion the poem was entitled "Our Group" signifying a sense of cohesion and intimacy. Feelings were more openly expressed and group member interaction was accelerated. Members exhibited mutual concern through the collaborative poem and an investment in the group.

Fifth Session

In this session, issues of honesty and individual freedoms emerged. Members continued to discuss the effect of depression on their interpersonal relationships and personal goals. Dan Hill's song "Sometimes When We Touch" was utilized to deal with some of the pain in communicating on an intimate level. Group members developed mutual support while each person continued to self-disclose. The collaborative poem reflected a greater sense of cohesion while each member worked towards differentiation.

Loose Ends
Feeling suspended in air
Vulnerable, uncertain
Every question raises a few more
something stuck in my throat
    as I dash for a finish line
    that I can't see
Closing off the passage ways
            of the maze
and risking new and old directions.
Meeting my other self . . .
    Turning my back on the closed
            passage ways.
    While I'm looking over my shoulder
    Yes, a sense of regret - a tearful hurt
            But
there's a fulfillment in our own abilities
to answer our own questions

Indeed the loose ends could be recognized and accepted. Rather than an obsession with the uncertainties, members could deal with problems in a constructive manner. With the end of group treatment becoming increasingly more apparent, group members were becoming more active. They were developing a sense of power and control over their own lives. Subsequently depressive behaviors were reduced.

Sixth Session

Perceptions of relationships appeared to be the dominant theme of this session. One single female talked about a relationship she was having with a married male. She had ambivalent feelings about continuing the relationship and sought feedback from the group. Although group members were cautious on the matter, they related to the struggle. Members discussed "ideal relationships" and the difficulties of finding a mate. Dan Hill's song "Perfect Man" was utilized to further develop the group's concerns. It contains the following lyrics. "I saw you as whatever dream / I wanted you to be / But I never saw you as a real person / The way you wanted to be seen." Issues of perceptions and meeting personal needs were included in the discussion.

The collaborative poem was entitled "Games." It again reflected the theme of the session and indicated the universality of feeling.

> Games
> We all play games with ourselves
> as well as with others
>   . . .
> we are the game
> we decide
> we play the game
> we survive
>   . . .

The group was working into the final stage of separation and exhibited some regressive behavior with a superficial discussion of relationships and perhaps a denial of group ending, as termination was to be the following week (e.g., "we decide . . . we survive").

Final Session

Richard Aldington's poem "New Love" was used in this final session to help deal with issues of termination and separation. This poem deals with pain as a part of growth. Cashman and West's song entitled "Lifesong" also proved helpful. Note the following lines: "And they say it would be so easy for me / If I accepted what I see with my eyes, / But I can't help blinking and I won't stop thinking /

Or looking for another side.'' These words provided a sense of validation and determination for the group. The following words brought them together again before they were to leave: "And don't we all fit together somehow / Or is it only just me? / Is anyone home or am I sailing alone / In my own little part of the sea? / . . . Life, sit down and talk with me / I've got some things to say.'' Indeed group members had found their voice and were able to act on their thoughts and feelings.

There was difficulty for group members to agree on the title of the collaborative poem. They finally decided:

> Group
> no real answers
> trying not to build a wall
> so high that we can't see over
> but high enough
> to protect our soft spots
> looking for friends
> with whom we can share our soft spots
> loving
> is being vulnerable
> we alternate
> between building up
> and tearing down our walls
>   . . .

This poem provided closure for the group. They recognized the continuing struggle between wanting to remain in a safe place and wanting to experience growth. They were in more control and could continue the search if they wished. Termination became a discussion of both finished and unfinished work within a time frame. Both group treatment and poetry are defined within boundaries; however, both remain timeless and unfinished. The client completes the poem or treatment session in his or her own time and space. The group can be just a beginning.

Discussion

The use of poetry and pop music was helpful in stimulating group interaction and treating the interpersonal aspects of depression. This is especially helpful in considering the low energy level of depressed clients. Of particular note, the use of poetry and music was helpful in accelerating or decelerating the pace of a session. In essence the rhythm of a poem or melody of a song could affect time in a therapeutic way. Many of the members were preoccupied with negative thoughts and self-defeating behaviors (e.g., "I'm worthless," or "I might as well stay at home"). Through poetry and/or music, the group leaders were able to reach members through cognitive processes which subsequently had impact on affective and behavioral processes. The poem and/or song seemed to quickly tap into the affective realm of individuals, bringing feelings to the surface. For example, one member verbalized that he wanted to be left alone. A song entitled "So You Couldn't Get to Me" was played. This stimulated group discussion and subsequently this quiet member began to reveal some painful experiences. Towards the end of the session he became the recorder for the collaborative poem (i.e., he got out of his seat and wrote down the lines), thus increasing his commitment and energy level and helping many other members feel connected. The poetry and music were also helpful in universalizing many of the feelings clients experienced (e.g., "Brooding—we will never be good enough to each other"). The use of poetry and music was helpful in bringing some members from a preoccupation with time past to an active stance in time present.

The timing of the collaborative poems (i.e., toward the end of each session) in which members worked together, appeared to advance group cohesion at a rather rapid pace. Providing copies of the members' collaborative poem in subsequent weeks also helped provide continuity between sessions. One especially interesting finding was the similarity between content of the collaborative poems and group developmental stages. In considering Garland et al. (1965) stages of group development, the following can be noted:

Week 1—*Pre-affiliation*: "inside a sinkhole / dark, grasping / don't want to do anything."

Week 2—*Power and Control*: "Anger/throwing stones at the moon / energy not directed well."

Week 3—*Intimacy*: "relief / is voicing / what you've been afraid to say."

Week 4—*Intimacy*: "delving into each other's feelings / . . . struggling with the cloud / grabbing each other."

Week 5—*Differentiation*: "there's a fulfillment in our own abilities / to answer our own questions."

Week 6—*Separation*: "empty interactions / a waste of time
. . . games are a way of life / a way to survive."
Week 7—*Separation/Termination*: "Our Group / undecided
about my feelings / but a little bit better equipped to share."

This may suggest that the collaborative poem, although an imposed structure on the group, did not impede but rather enhanced and accelerated group development. This technique was especially helpful in the time limited modality (i.e., 7 weeks) by quickly involving members in a concrete shared experience thus advancing cohesion.

The use of poetry and/or music in group treatment has limitations and requires a careful assessment of group development and individual needs before being utilized. The timing and amount of time spent using poetic techniques is especially important. To be effective, the poetic material must be seen by the group as connected to their processes. This can prompt here-and-now discussion; however, too much time can be spent on a poem or song. Some poems or songs may be aversive to members or evoke feelings he or she might not be ready to encounter. In instances when this happens, the variable of time itself can be helpful. Through the leader or through group forces the individual could be supported with the notion that she/he had control over the use of time and was free to choose not to deal with those feelings at that time. This type of decision provides a boundary for feelings and may restore a sense of independence.

Poems or songs can also provide a means to remain withdrawn (i.e., escape). It is perhaps especially important to observe (e.g., nonverbal behaviors) the effect on more silent members. This is one area when it is especially helpful to have co-leaders. The use of pre-existing poems can inadvertently force rather than facilitate group process if group leaders are determined to use a poem or song in a given session, perhaps serving the needs of the leader(s) rather than the members. The intention of this poetic technique is to facilitate not substitute for group content and process. This perspective avoids a literary or educational emphasis.

Poetry and music appear to have potential as ancillary therapeutic group techniques. They are not considered therapeutic entities in this report. Poetry and music are especially helpful in working with clients at a university counseling center by enhancing *early* engagement in short-term group treatment through a nonthreatening medium. The collaborative poems were instrumental in advancing group cohesion and served as a form of ritual for termination. The collab-

orative poems were useful in connecting sessions, but more importantly, in connecting people in a relatively brief period of time. For
the group leader(s) who is (are) comfortable in a facilitative stance
with the use of the arts, poetry and music are additional techniques
that may prove valuable in reaching cognitive, affective and behavioral domains and subsequently advancing group process.

By relating to and taking strength from personally meaningful
poetry or music, group members were able to reduce dependency on
the group leaders. Group members found methods to deal with
depression and other problems from within themselves and through
each other. The poems or song lyrics provided the necessary boundaries or structure for what were sometimes confusing and ambivalent feelings. The final collaborative poem includes a review of
boundaries: "building up / and tearing down walls" and the willingness to risk "looking for friends / with whom we can share our soft
spots."

The group treatment session constitutes only a fragment of a
client's week. Through the use of time, poetry and music the group
leader(s) can help clients maximize their therapeutic experience and
create the means for progress beyond the session. The structure,
measure and movement of time, poetry and music were most compatible with group processes and treatment goals of the aforemen-
tioned group. It is perhaps a reminder of the art of group work practice.

REFERENCES

Boyum, R. (1978). Therapeutic uses of pop music. *Journal of College Student Personnel, 19,*
    363.
Bresler, E. (1982). Filling an empty universe: Poetry therapy with a group of emotionally
    isolated men. *Social Work with Groups, 5*(3), 65-70.
Buck, L. A., & Kramer, A. (1974). Poetry as a means of group facilitation. *Journal of
    Humanistic Psychology, 14*(1), 57-71.
Davis, M. S. (1979). Poetry therapy versus interpersonal group therapy: Comparison of
    treatment effectiveness with depressed women (Doctoral dissertation, The Wright In-
    stitute, 1978). *Dissertation Abstracts International, 39,* 5543B.
Derogatis, L. R. (1978). Brief Hopkins Psychiatric Rating Scale.
Edgar, K. F., & Hazley, F. (1969). Validation of poetry as a group therapy technique. In
    J. J. Leedy (Ed.), *Poetry therapy* (pp. 111-123). Philadelphia: J. B. Lippincott.
Garland, J. A., Jones, H., & Kolodny, R. (1965). A model for stages of development in
    social work groups. In S. Bernstein (Ed.), *Explorations in group work* (pp. 12-53).
    Boston: Boston University School of Social Work.
Lauer, R., & Goldfield, M. (1970). Creative writing in group therapy. *Psychotherapy:
    Theory, Research, and Practice, 7*(4), 248-252.

Leedy, J. J. (1969). Principles of poetry therapy. In J. J. Leedy (Ed.), *Poetry therapy* (pp. 67-74). Philadelphia: J. B. Lippincott.

Lerner, A. (1982). Poetry therapy in the group experience. In L. E. Abt & I. R. Stuart (Eds.), *The newer therapies: A sourcebook* (pp. 228-248). New York: Van Nostrand Reinhold.

Lessner, J. W. (1974). The poem as catalyst in group counseling. *Personnel and Guidance Journal, 53*(2), 33-38.

Mazza, N. (1979). Poetry: A therapeutic tool in the early stages of alcoholism treatment. *Journal of Studies on Alcohol, 40*(1), 123-128.

Mazza, N. (1981). The use of poetry in treating the troubled adolescent. *Adolescence, 16* (62), 403-408.

Mazza, N. (1981). Poetry and group counseling: An exploratory study (Doctoral dissertation, The Florida State University, 1981). *Dissertation Abstracts International, 42*(6).

Mazza, N., & Prescott, B. (1981). Poetry: An ancillary technique in couples group therapy. *American Journal of Family Therapy, 9*(1), 53-57.

Ross, D. L. (1977). Poetry therapy versus traditional supportive therapy: A comparison of group process (Doctoral dissertation, Case Western Reserve University, 1977). *Dissertation Abstracts International, 38,* 1417B-1418B.

Santiago, P. R. (1969). The lyrical expression of adolescent conflict in Beatles songs. *Adolescence, 4,* 199-210.

Williams, J. (1978). The effectiveness of poetry in facilitating openness (Doctoral dissertation, Purdue University, 1978). *Dissertation Abstracts International, 39,* 4603B.

Poems

Aldington, R. Epigrams (New love). In W. Pratt (Ed.), *The imagist poem* (p. 73). New York: E. P. Dutton.

Crane, S. If I should cast off this tattered coat. In A. Dore (Ed.), *The premier book of major poets* (p. 288). Greenwich, CT: Fawcett.

Ignatow, D. Brooding. In *Figures of the human.* Middletown, CT: Wesleyan University Press.

Songs

Cashman, T., & West, T. (1974). *Lifesong.* Sweet City Songs, Inc.

Fox, C., & Gimble, N. (1973). *I got a name.* Fox Fanfare Music.

Hill, D. (1979). *Perfect man.* If Dreams Had Wings Music Ltd.

Hill, D., & Mann, B. (1977). *Sometimes when we touch.* Welbeck Music (ASCAP) and ATV Music BMI.

Loggins, D. (1974). *So you couldn't get to me.* Leeds Music Corp./Antique Music (ASCAP).

Patterns of Entry and Exit
in Open-Ended Groups

Maeda J. Galinsky
Janice H. Schopler

ABSTRACT. This descriptive study of 66 open-ended groups identifies characteristics and patterns found in open group systems. While the groups endure over time, members typically stay for only brief periods. Membership change, the dominant feature of these groups, is associated with the frequent use of systematic procedures for member entry and exit. These procedures, designed to maintain group stability and speed member integration, offer useful guidance to practitioners coping with ongoing and often unpredictable change in open-ended groups.

Introduction

Open-ended groups represent a unique time perspective. The group system endures over time, but the tenure of individual members is typically brief. The open-ended group is designed to offer an immediate, ongoing response to client needs; members can enter and depart on a continuous basis without waiting until a new group is formed. The time-limited pattern of membership is determined by several factors. Length of stay may be dictated by the focus of the group, as in orientation groups; by the boundaries of contact with an agency, as in groups for parents of hospitalized children; by fulfillment of a court order, as in groups for spouse

Maeda J. Galinsky, PhD, is Professor, and Janice H. Schopler, ACSW, is Associate Professor at the School of Social Work, University of North Carolina, 223 E. Franklin Street 150 A, Chapel Hill, North Carolina 27514.

The research reported in this paper was supported by a grant from the University Research Council of the University of North Carolina at Chapel Hill. The authors appreciate this support and also wish to thank the many practitioners who responded to our questionnaire; our research assistant, Patricia McGarry; our computer programmer, Kenneth W. Yow; and our colleague and consultant, H. Carl Henley, Jr. These results were originally presented at the Fifth Annual Symposium for the Advancement of Social Work with Groups, Detroit, Michigan, October 21, 1983.

abusers; by achievement of personal goals, as in therapy groups for mothers of preschool children; or, by temporary member need for crisis counseling and support, as in groups for relatives of newly diagnosed Alzheimer's disease patients. While some members contract beforehand for the number of sessions they will attend, the period of participation is often unpredictable, either because member relationships with the organization are variable, or because some members achieve their purposes more rapidly than others.

Because of the frequent turnover, circumscribed stay and unpredictability of membership, there is a need to focus quickly on the task to ensure that members receive the services intended. Members know their time together may be brief. Some members may come for only one session and many attend less than five meetings.[1] For current members to see results, each session must be productive.

A constant feature of open-ended groups is the ever-present possibility of member entry or exit. While frequency of membership change varies, each time a new member is added or an old one leaves, the group must adapt to the change in composition. At the same time that open membership provides a necessary flexibility, it also leads to a disruption of the group process and creates a challenge for the practitioner, requiring new conceptual and practice tools to cope with these perpetual changes.

The questions of practitioners seeking more effective ways to contend with continual member entry and exit prompted our interest in this research. Seeking answers, we reviewed the literature and found extensive reports of varied practitioner experiences with open-ended groups but few theoretical discussions. Existing group theory tends to focus on groups with stable long-term membership and provides little direction for interventions to support ongoing membership change.[2] Disparate accounts from practice did, however, provide a basis for our beginning conceptualization of open-ended groups. We identified the purposes, composition, group arrangements, group development, structure and processes found in the open-ended groups reported in the literature and offered guidelines for intervention (Schopler and Galinsky, 1984).

In this descriptive study of open-ended groups, we are exploring patterns and interventions associated with open membership and the validity of the principles we suggested. The empirical description of current practice is intended to provide a beginning base for the development of theory supporting practitioner efforts. Since our data collection is still in process, we are reporting our preliminary findings as they relate to group characteristics and patterns of member entry and departure and to the practitioner interventions used to deal with membership change. At a later date we will be examining the relationships among patterns, interventions and the course of group development in our expanded sample.

Method of Study

Our data are derived from questionnaires completed by social work practitioners about the open-ended groups they lead or co-lead. Open-ended groups are defined by the intent to keep membership open, whether change occurs every meeting or as infrequently as once in six months. To locate respondents, we are polling current and recent field instructors of the School of Social Work of the University of North Carolina by telephone to determine if they are serving open-ended groups and to obtain names of other practitioners leading such groups. The sample to date includes a wide range of groups served in both public and private agencies in central North Carolina.

Respondents are asked to complete a questionnaire designed to elicit information about group purpose, composition, group arrangements, entry of new members, termination of old members, and group development. Further, respondents are asked to give their impressions of the advantages and disadvantages related to open membership in groups and to describe any special procedures they find helpful in their work.

Description of the Respondents

The 55 social workers who completed the questionnaires included in our preliminary analysis represent a total of 66 open-ended groups. The 89% response rate is only tentative since there has not been sufficient time for all questionnaires to be completed and we are still soliciting respondents. Forty-five individuals reported on one group; nine reported on two groups; and, one respondent reported on three groups. Three-fourths of the 55 respondents are direct service workers and about three-fifths of them work at inpatient or residential settings. A slight majority of the respondents are in the field of Mental Health but other areas, such as Health, Family and Children, and Aging are also included. Most of these social workers are in settings where the primary focus is on the provision of clinical services with a few in outreach and training organizations or in agencies combining these two functions.

All of the respondents were trained social workers who had at least an MSW, except for one person with a PhD who co-led a group with an MSW. They tended to be experienced practitioners who had some type of formal preparation for group work either through their social work education or other types of training.

Description of the Sample

The current sample consists of 66 groups, all led or co-led by social work professionals. These groups may not be representative of all open-ended groups, but they exemplify the range of groups formed to serve people who have pressing needs on an ongoing basis. They include groups for cancer patients who need continuing support, education about the disease, and coping skills to meet the often devastating consequences for their personal, family, and work lives; groups for adolescents living in group homes who have to deal with issues of group living, of identity, and of family relationships; groups of chronically mentally ill residing in the community and learning to deal with a non-institutional setting, with interpersonal problems, with "dead time" and with the response of others to their condition; and, groups to provide support and help to caregivers in nursing homes, where demanding and sometimes tedious tasks often cause stress and boredom. The groups we examined were located in mental hospitals, general hospitals, community mental health centers, half-way houses for mental patients, group care facilities for youth, child abuse prevention programs and family service agencies, to name but a few. Despite the diversity of these groups, they all have open boundaries and deal with membership change on a continuing basis.

Purposes

The majority of the groups examined were created to provide services to adults, with some groups serving children and adolescents, and a few serving a mixture of both. Most groups were directed to the identified client, whether that was the sole emphasis or also involved significant others in the clients' lives. A few were for significant others only or for staff. Family and individual problems were the primary focus in the majority (59%) of these groups; the remainder of the groups had a primary focus on lack of interpersonal/ task/social skills (18%), need for information (15%), group living issues (5%) and job-stress related problems (3%).

Whatever their primary focus, the groups in our sample addressed a multiplicity of specific purposes to meet member needs. Responses to a checklist of ten possible purposes indicated that 41% of the groups held six or more of these purposes, 45% of the groups held four or five purposes, and 14% addressed two or three purposes. Not a single group was designed to meet only one purpose. The specific purposes were checked with variable frequency: support (94%), problem-solving (88%), education (76%), training for staff and students (68%), treatment (64%), skills training (53%), orientation (36%), advocacy (20%), screening and assessment (18%), and other, including aims such as coordination of services (8%).

Composition

Leadership patterns indicated a predominance of co-leaders: 88% of the groups were led by two or more practitioners. Group size is fairly constant and falls within a narrow range for most groups: 76% of the groups reported an average attendance of 4, 5, 6, or 7 members, with a modal response of 5. Almost all groups could identify such an average attendance. Workers reported that there was considerable variation in attendance from meeting to meeting in about half of the groups, while the other half reported little variation. Of those 35 groups which experienced fluctuations, over half noted that they could expect differences in size of between 1 and 5 persons from meeting to meeting. A modal response of 8 members (26%) was reported for greatest number attending; most groups (70%) had anywhere from 6 to 10 members as their highest attendance.

Potential members were drawn from a number of sources. Members came from staff referrals, from the workers' caseloads, from self-referral, or from advertisements. In addition, members were referred by professionals in related organizations; or, were invited to attend because of their particular status (e.g., parent of child in the project, cancer patient, resident).

Not all potential members were accepted into the groups in the sample; about three-fifths had some type of criteria for member selection or exclusion, and some respondents used multiple criteria to determine membership. Criteria used to screen potential members included: common diagnosis or problem; selected characteristics such as age, marital status, and sex; compatibility with current membership; severity of problematic condition; and other considerations such as motivation to attend and agency priorities. When members were accepted for the group, respondents viewed attendance as voluntary in slightly over half of the groups, required in 26%, and a mixture in 21%.

Group Arrangements

Group meetings varied from once a week in 44% of the groups, the most typical pattern, to no established pattern in one group. The remaining groups met anywhere from every day to less than once a month. The length of meetings showed little variation from usual group practice. In half of the groups, meetings were one hour or less; most of the rest met for between 61 minutes and two hours.

The overwhelming majority (77%) of these groups had been in existence for two years or more. Only 9% of the groups had met for less than a year. In 55% of the groups, members were asked to make a commitment to attend for either a specific number of sessions (ranging from 1 to 24 meetings) or for all of the sessions offered while they were identified clients or during their residence in an inpatient facility. In groups requiring no commitment, attendance appeared to be based solely on member need and motivation.

For the 35 groups in which an average attendance rate could be identified, there was wide variation in the typical number of sessions attended. In many (71%) of these groups, membership was relatively short-term, with estimates of average attendance ranging from one to ten sessions. In less than a third (29%) of these groups, membership tended to be longer-term and average attendance ranged from eleven to fifty sessions. For the other 31 groups in the sample, no standard pattern of attendance could be identified.

Entry Patterns

The theme of variation continues in the patterns of member entry reported for our sample of open-ended groups. Members were added almost every meeting in 29% of the groups, every two to four meetings in 20%, every five to ten meetings in 18%, and at intervals greater than ten meetings for 5%. For 29% of the groups, the timing of member additions was variable within each of the groups. The number of members added at one time was predominantly one (41%) or two (24%). In an additional 5% of the groups, either 4, 5, or 14 members were typically added at one time. About one-third of the groups had developed no pattern for the number of member additions.

Exit Patterns

Exit patterns for members of the open-ended groups studied are even more variable than those related to entry. In 38% of the groups there was no pattern related to how often members left. In the remaining groups, members left almost every meeting in 20% of the groups, every two to four meetings in 20%, every five to ten in 20%, and only after more than ten meetings in 2%. The number of members leaving at one time was not predictable in 41% of the groups, was reported as one member in 42%, two members in 16%, and three members in 2% of the groups.

Procedures for Entry

Given the potential for disruption created by members entering the groups in the sample in an often unpredictable fashion, it is not surprising that all but two of the groups (97%) had procedures for handling member entry. Response to a checklist of possible procedures indicated that in 62% of the groups employing procedures pre-group interviews were used, 89% of the groups had verbal orientation, 27% used structured exercises and activities, and 12% used other introductory mechanisms like taking a group pledge. Procedures were most often used in combination, with two-thirds of the groups using two or more of these procedures.

In slightly more than two-thirds of the groups, the group members were involved with the worker in orienting new members. In the remaining groups, workers took total responsibility for this task and occasionally involved other personnel. The most common means of orienting new members was the presentation of group purposes; this occurred in almost all of the groups (98%). Introduction of new members (91%) and the presentation of rules or norms (84%) were also very frequent approaches and over half (56%) included presentation of member responsibilities. Further, in 20% of the groups other means were used such as previewing the group or reviewing group history. Usually more than one approach was taken to orientation; four-fifths of the groups reporting their approach to orientation used three or more of the five means cited. Only two groups used one means alone.

Procedures for Termination

In contrast to the pervasive use of entry procedures by almost all of the sample, somewhat fewer groups reported established procedures to deal with member termination: 71% had procedures while 29% reported no procedures. Responses to a checklist of possible exit procedures indicate that group discussion related to termination issues and evaluation was a procedure used in most of the groups (91%). Structured exercises or activities (32%), post-group interviews (23%) and other procedures (28%) such as provision of refreshments were used less frequently. In slightly less than one-half of the groups only one procedure was used, while a combination of procedures was employed in the other groups.

As with entry, responsibility for handling termination was most commonly shared by workers and members (72%). In some groups (23%) the workers handled termination alone and there was one instance reported of members taking sole responsibility for termination and one group where responsibility was carried by other personnel outside the group.

All of the groups reporting termination procedures included review of achievements and expression of feelings as means to deal with member departure. Most groups also discussed members' future plans (94%) and a number of groups (32%) had additional means of dealing with members leaving such as requiring advance notice of member departure or focusing on unfinished business. Multiple means were uniformly used to deal with termination.

Discussion

The large number of open-ended groups located in a small geographic area indicates that open membership is becoming a relatively common feature of groups designed by seasoned practitioners. A majority of these open-ended groups appear to be an established and accepted part of agency services and do not represent an experimental venture.[3] It should be noted that our sample of open-ended groups was provided by practitioners with professional education in social work, experience, and considerable training in group approaches. These social workers have adapted their knowledge and skills in a way that facilitates responsive service delivery in a wide range of settings. The open-ended groups they have created provide ongoing service to adults, adolescents and children with needs related to mental health, aging, family and interpersonal relations, and health.

Despite the varied client populations served, these groups held many purposes in common and typically were designed to meet a multiplicity of needs, an indicator of their versatility and flexibility. They tended to meet on a regular basis and to share common group experiences stemming from the unpredictability and disruption associated with open membership. While there was considerable range in the number of sessions attended, the predominant mode was short-term attendance. Given the uncertain and brief nature of membership, workers may find it helpful to have a number of purposes available so that they can be responsive to those present and quickly focus their work together. The groups in our sample did exhibit a variety of patterns. They differed in size, frequency of meetings, requirements of attendance, criteria for membership, source of members, as well as the frequency and amount of membership change.

The primary identifying characteristic of open-ended groups is that of membership change: over time, old members depart and new members are added, sometimes in the same session. Because turnover was fairly frequent in the groups in the sample, entry and exit were common themes. While the number of individuals involved in membership change was typically small, entry and exit still constitute disruption of group activities. Just as constant turnover affects a group and its members, groups that experience continuity for longer periods may react even more strongly to the introduction of a new member or loss of an old. These groups may have had more opportunity to develop cohesion and lower expectations for change in membership.

In many of the groups there was a certain degree of unpredictability related to the arrival of new members and the departure of old. A sizeable minority of the groups studied had no definable pattern related to the timing of membership changes. Further, since only slightly more than half of the groups had requirements for attendance, practitioners often were unaware of how many members would be present at any given session. Thus, changes in membership disrupting the flow of group life and some unpredictability are expected features in these open-ended groups.

Established procedures for orienting new members and handling termination of members who are leaving can minimize potential disruption to the group and offset unpredictability. This is especially critical since members of open-ended groups often attend for only a short time. Almost all of the groups had procedures related to member entry and almost three-fourths had a standard approach for dealing with termination. Perhaps termination procedures were less developed because members often left without advance notice. Workers and members may have had no further contact with them. In contrast, new arrivals had to be oriented whether or not they were anticipated.

Although procedures for termination are not used as frequently as those for entry, their development merits consideration. Old members need to express feelings related to loss, envy, abandonment, or pride in others' accomplishments, to facilitate reintegration as they proceed with their work together. Even when members are only in the group for a brief period, there should be an opportunity to reflect on the experience and to evaluate its impact. Further, when turnover is rapid, termination routines can give a sense of stability to the group. Termination procedures have a way of signaling to the remaining members that each individual is important to the group's life and will be missed on departure, reinforcing the importance of the group. Even members who do not return to the group for termination may be contacted, in person, by phone, or in writing, to review their time with the group.

Workers and members most often shared responsibility for entry and exit routines. While group workers strive to have members take responsibility for group functioning, there may not be sufficient time for leadership to emerge in groups where members come for brief periods. Thus, it may be necessary for the worker to assume some leadership role in entry and exit, involving the members as much as possible. Practitioners used a variety of approaches to orient new members and speed integration, including both discussion and structured activities. They described a number of innovative techniques for connecting new members to old and providing continuity to group purposes and traditions. Many of the rituals were designed to convey information about the group and the potential help it could offer. New members were sometimes given a written description, allowed to preview sessions on video tape or as observers, greeted with songs or welcome cards, offered refreshments or assigned a "buddy." Old members often reviewed their goals and needs and assisted newcomers in defining their stake in the group. These varied traditions not only help integrate new members into the group system, but also ease tension for the rest of the group by providing a structured way to deal with an ever-changing situation. The reaffirmation of goals, norms, and mutual interests that are a product of these procedures can be a renewing force. Since these procedures typically are routinized, the group can move quickly through the necessary beginning tasks minimizing the boredom that might result from frequent repetition.

Even though entry tended to be handled in a most systematic way than termination, provision was made in a large number of the groups for departing members to examine and consolidate their group experience and for the remaining members to reassess and continue with their work together. Discussion may include reminiscence, evaluation of progress, exploration of future plans and available support systems, and expressions of loss. When termination was anticipated, many groups had some special way of wishing departing members well and celebrating their gains, sometimes through tangible means such as parties, cards, remembrance booklets, legacy tapes and awards. In one children's group, members previewed each member's departure in a symbolic train ride; and, several groups indicated that ritual activities and discussions were conducted with those remaining even when members had departed unexpectedly. In a number of cases, open membership implied ongoing availability of group support and when this was true, members who left were encouraged to return if they wished.

The procedures used to cope with entry and exit in this sample of open-ended groups tend to reinforce the value of the group and promote stability despite frequent change. Workers may not be able to anticipate new arrivals or sudden departures, but routine responses to these events can reduce the uncertainty of open membership and allay the negative impact of change. We would recommend that every group develop systematic procedures for dealing with member entry and departure. These procedures should address not only the needs of new arrivals and members who are leaving but should also encompass the group's need to reintegrate after every membership change.

Practitioners responding to our questionnaire have developed a broad array of means for dealing with the disruptive effect of membership turnover despite a lack of theoretical and practice guidelines. They cope creatively with constant change, using entry and exit rituals to ease the work of the group as members enter and

leave. Their responses represent practice adaptations of theory pertaining to closed groups.

The time-limited membership often characteristic of open-ended
groups must be considered in both group composition and orientation. In the majority of groups in the sample, some type of inclusion
or exclusion criteria were used to recruit and select members with
common interests, a practice which should expedite rapid group formation and effective group functioning. The fact that membership
was regarded as completely voluntary in over half of the groups
and partially voluntary in an additional one-fifth may reflect the
workers' recognition that members must be motivated to accomplish
their goals in a limited period of time. Furthermore, the requirement
that members commit themselves to attendance for a prescribed
number of sessions in slightly over half of the groups may speak to
the attempt to bring some stability and predictability to a group
situation constantly in flux.

Working with open-ended groups demands a high level of skill,
knowledge, and flexibility. To achieve the purposes for which their
groups are formed, practitioners must continually and instantly
assess individual and group behavior and respond to ever-changing
situations. They must be ready to alter plans to accommodate to un-
anticipated membership turnover or unforeseen crises. They must
be skilled in a variety of approaches so that they can be responsive to
the members present at any particular session. They must be able to
foster the rapid development of relationships which facilitate the
achievement of members' goals. Sometimes, workers may need to
be directive to keep groups moving, to fill vacuums created by
membership loss, and to ensure that group purposes and maintenance needs are given adequate attention; at other times, when
members are able to perform leadership functions, the worker must
be prepared to take a less active role.

These practitioners must also fend off the tedium that comes with
constant repetition. Since members come for limited periods, entry
and exit must be encountered over and over, creating the potential
for worker boredom and burnout. Additionally, group workers may
be involved in training students and other co-workers in the open-
ended approach. These taxing leadership demands may explain, to
some extent, why the vast majority of open-ended groups are served
by two or more co-leaders. Co-leadership is one way to secure support and cope with the difficulties and frustrations these groups may
entail.

Since new members continually enter open-ended groups and old members depart, the formation and termination phases of group development are perpetually repeated, even if only for a brief period each time. When members remain in groups for longer intervals, the initial or formative phase of development may occur through a gradual build-up to the next phase; in the time-limited atmosphere of the open-ended group this process must be telescoped. Similarly, as termination occurs frequently, and sometimes without warning, leaders must be prepared to adapt their knowledge of termination guidelines to take account of members' often brief stays and the group's need to proceed with its work.

Our preliminary analysis of this sample of 66 open-ended groups suggests that open membership has become a standard feature of group services. Most of the groups in our sample had been in operation for several years, a testament to their ability to attract members on a continuing basis. The procedures practitioners have developed tend to maintain group stability and integration in the face of unpredictable and sometimes disruptive membership change. While we do not have any evidence indicating that these groups accomplish all the purposes they pursue, we have data which suggest many groups move beyond the initial stages of group development. Further, the longevity of these groups and the statements of our respondents affirm the importance of open-ended groups in meeting members' needs.

The frequent use of open-ended groups by trained and skilled practitioners warrants further examination and research. Open membership deserves increased conceptual attention. Practitioners who are demonstrating the utility and flexibility of open-ended groups in a variety of settings offer an ample data base for describing critical features of this approach and for developing theory to guide intervention.

NOTES

1. Although brief membership is the prototype for open-ended groups, members in some open-ended therapy groups may remain for two years or longer. In certain groups, members may leave and then return as often and for as long as they wish.

2. Very recently, principles related to open-ended groups have begun to appear in the group literature. See especially: Irvin D. Yalom, *Inpatient Group Psychotherapy* (New York: Basic Books, Inc., 1983), pp. 74-82; and, Sue Henry, *Group Skills in Social Work* (Itasca, IL: F. E. Peacock Publishers, Inc., 1981), pp. 301-318.

3. In a recent collection of articles describing short-term therapy groups, more than one-half the chapters were devoted to groups with open membership. See Max Rosenbaum (ed.), *Handbook of Short-Term Therapy Groups* (New York: McGraw-Hill Book Co., 1983).

REFERENCE

Schopler, J. H. & Galinsky, M. J. (1984). Meeting practice needs: Conceptualizing the open-ended group. *Social Work with Groups, 7* (Summer), 3-21; also (in press). The open-ended group. In *Individual Change through Small Groups* (2nd ed.), Paul H. Glasser and Martin Sundel. New York: The Free Press.

On the Potentiality
and Limits of Time:
The Single-Session Group
and the Cancer Patient

Lisa Rae Block

ABSTRACT. Although use of the single-session group is increasing, specific research remains minimal. Since traditional models of group work do not seem to adequately conceptualize these groups, the intent of this paper is to present a beginning *handbook* for the single-session worker. The single-session group will be examined as it both follows and departs from general group work theory. Explored will be the ramifications of these departures for framework, group structure, process, phasic development, goals and worker's role. Alternate formats will be discussed and recommendations for practice outlined. Focus is the use of these groups in an acute-care hospital specialized in the treatment of cancer patients.

The single-session group is no ordinary group. To lead one presents a challenge to even the most seasoned practitioner. Some social workers question whether these *one-shot deals* should be called *groups* at all. The groups to be discussed here are those offered to the patients at Memorial Sloan-Kettering Cancer Center to provide information and mutual support and help them cope with their cancer. But do they also present them, in an ironic way, with an additional "existential dilemma?" Likewise for staff, supervisors, social work practice and theory, these single-session groups basically remain an enigma. Can they be done? Are they real?

The *reality* and usefulness of the single-session group are basic assumptions of this paper. In fact, one of its goals is to help legiti-

Lisa Rae Block, MSW, CSW, is a social worker in the In-patient Neuro/Neurosurgery unit, Memorial Sloan-Kettering Cancer Center, New York. The background for this paper was the experience gained by the author as a student intern at Memorial Sloan-Kettering Cancer Center, during the academic year 1982-1983.

mate such groups within the social work profession, both to increase worker effectiveness and personal satisfaction and to encourage the much needed research focus. The issue here is not one of *existence.* The single-session is possible and a valid group type. Rather, the issue is one of quality. What makes for a *good enough* single-session group?

Although use of the single-session group is increasing, specific research remains minimal. The task at hand, then, is to present a model and offer an approach that will address the ''how.'' The goal is to suggest guidelines for intervention, and a perspective that will aid in understanding, appreciating and, perhaps, even predicting the dynamics of the single-session group. The end result will, hopefully, be a beginning *handbook* for the single-session worker.

The single-session group will be examined as it both follows and departs from general groupwork theory. What will be explored are the ramifications of its time-limited nature for conceptual framework, group structure, process, phasic development, goals and worker's role. Alternate formats for such groups will be discussed and recommendations for practice outlined. The model proposed will, ideally, be applicable to a variety of settings. But the main focus of both the literature review and discussion is the use of these single-session groups with cancer patients, particularly those who are hospitalized.

Definition: What Is a Single-Session Group?

A group can be defined as two or more persons in face-to-face contact interacting around a commonality over time, *however brief* (Schwartz, 1968; Casper, 1981). Social work practice with a group is neither dependent on any particular time line nor any particular group purpose(s). In the single-session group, ''the particular collectivity comes together for this particular purpose only once'' (Casper, 1981, pp. 2, 13).

The single-session group for cancer patients can be seen as a type of *situation/transition* group (Schwartz, 1975). It offers information, social support, and opportunity to interact with others who share a similar life stress (Robinovitch and Ransohoff, 1981, p. 61).

For the most part, the single-session educational/support groups at Memorial Hospital meet once a week. Since length of hospital stay is usually seven to ten days, it is usually not the case that a patient will be hospitalized long enough to attend more than one such group. If hospitalization is for a longer period it is often due to medical complications, in which case the patient's physical condition would probably preclude attendance. On some of the units, patient groups meet more than once a week. Examples are the preparatory pre-surgical groups for patients with lung cancer and the rehabilitative post-mastectomy groups for those with breast cancer (Euster, 1979). But even here, membership (and size) varies from session to session due to admissions and discharges, operating room and other hospital schedules, medical conditions and the like.

Although the function of such a group may remain the same and some people will attend more than once (or upon a subsequent admission), these are *open* groups by definition and by necessity. More often than not, this openness means an almost entirely new membership each session. Thus these groups are viewed as self-contained units, each with its own beginning, climax, and ending. They are not part of a larger whole, be it short- or long-term. Purpose and contract in a single-session need to be restated and renegotiated every time a group convenes. Any carryover by members from one session to the next is an unexpected bonus (Casper, 1981, p. 14); it should not be expected. The continuity that does exist, as will be suggested later, in part resides in the leaders themselves and the themes they help to extract in group process.

This then is the one-shot deal. It is a group for which some say there is no past and no future, and one whose lifetime is usually no more than 1-1/2 hours (Shalinsky, 1981, p. 9).

Time as an Independent Variable

For the Group

"The words TIME and PATIENCE must be written in capitalized letters in social group work," writes Gisela Konopka (1963, p. 159). Time looms as a significant factor in these single-session groups. They are short-term par excellence. And one must be sensitive, both in practice and theory, to the different time sense that is operating. ". . . (S)hort-term treatment is not just a small sample of what the client might be lucky to get more of. It is a different experience. . ." (p. vii). The worker must recognize the dynamics inherent in limits imposed by time as well as the inevitable limits within these dynamics (*ibid.*). Time constraints (Casper, 1981) need not have an inevitable deleterious effect. More is not always better.

It is a theme throughout this paper that within the short life-span of a single-session group exists the opportunity for both potential and limitation. These groups can be productive and worthwhile for both members and leaders. But proper attention must be given by the latter to the implications that this *condensation* has for recruitment, contract, structure, cohesion, closure and, most importantly, the worker's role in guiding group process through beginning, middle, and end phases.

The time-lapse quality of the process in single-session groups, like all short-term work, serves to remind the worker that time is always a factor and must also be a focus. There can be *telescoping* effect in a time-limited group. The knowledge of a limited duration may actually encourage a group to work and complete objectives more quickly and in less time than a group without such time limits (Hartford, 1971, p. 183; Schwartz, 1968).

These single-sessions also help to destroy the *illusion of unending time* so often found in long-term treatment. Terminations are not to be avoided. In fact, they remain the implicit goal of all therapeutic work. To the single-session worker, it soon becomes self-evident that termination is an issue that must begin with group contract.

For the Members

The characteristic loss of the perception of unending time that confronts an individual with cancer obligates him/her to learn to live in permanent uncertainty about the future (Rickert and Koffmann, 1982, p. 33). There is often a shift of priorities and an increased focus on the present. The increased awareness of the passage of time that accompanies learning to cope with cancer often seems to accelerate the process of personal growth (Spiegel and Yalom, 1978). Thus, the diagnosis of cancer can be said to have a telescoping effect for each patient. The single-session group (or any group) is by no means the only suggested mode of providing information and support to the patients in an acute-care hospital setting (Christ, 1982a). However, their generally high level of motivation and need tends to make them very receptive to the demands of the group's time limits. As in crisis groups, the time-limited single-session can offer benefits to its members that extent far beyond its temporal significance (Euster, 1979, p. 262).

Although cancer is no longer inevitably fatal, it does serve as a rather forceful reminder to all (patients, family, and staff) that lives are time-limited. "Cancer connects us to one another because having cancer is an embodiment of the existential paradox that we all experience: we feel we are immortal, yet we know that we will die" (Trillin, 1981, p. 699). Cancer undermines one's tacit assumption of immortality and his/her denial of death (Euster, 1979; Rickert and Koffmann, 1982; Becker, 1973).

Perhaps an analogy can be drawn here between the cancer patient and the single-session group. Both represent, in effect, an exaggeration of a reality. For both, time is never endless and purposes and goals need to be realistic.

To quote Carel Germain (1976):

> (T)ime (is) both the inevitable medium of human creativity and the symbol of the human being's final limitation . . . Time is the silent language that speaks of *potentiality and limits,* of creativity and death, of change and permanence. (pp. 419-20)[1]

What is further implied in this analogy is that what at first glance seems unique and different may, upon closer look, actually be a difference in order rather than kind. Working with a cancer patient can teach a professional a lot about him/herself. Running a single-session group can highlight for a worker many of the dynamics operating in all groups. The one-shot deal may be a different *animal,* but it is still of the same species.

Review of the Literature

If the single-session were to be classified a *rare* species, it would be more a comment on its special qualities than its lack of abundance. Its use is increasing in hospital settings, both medical and psychiatric, due to decreased lengths of stay and increased appreciation of the group mode (Lonergan, 1982). But in many ways the single-session has only recently been discovered by the social work profession. In fact, several of the most pertinent references cited here are unpublished papers (Casper, 1981; Crawford, 1982; Shalinsky, 1981).

There are no single-session classics. Although the works of Garland et al. (1973) on developmental phases and Yalom (1975) on curative factors and cohesiveness must be considered, adaptations are required before these concepts can be applied. As Shalinsky (1981) points out in his excellent survey, much of the background literature relevant to such a study must be drawn from many areas and from work, both short- and long-term, with individuals and groups. The task is then to integrate this material into a meaningful framework of practice.

The Setting

The various journal articles describing programs for oncology (and other) patients and their families emphasize the importance of conceptualizing the group, hospital unit, and each individual client as an intersection of various systems (Weiner, 1959; Dinerman et al., 1980; Christ, 1983). Leader confidence and group potential can depend on the institutionalization of the group into hospital routine and sanction into the medical complex (Lonergan, 1982, p. 30). The importance of systems work is particularly exaggerated in the case of the single-session group which largely derives its sense of continuity from the individual hospital unit (Shalinsky, 1981).

The element of *crisis* that can accompany any serious illness and/ or hospitalization (Falck, 1978; Lonergan, 1982) becomes intensified when the illness is that of cancer. The difficult issues that are raised and must be confronted by patients in such a setting, however, demand that the staff first must deal with *obstacles to the search for common ground* (Schwartz, 1961; Shulman, 1979) that exist among themselves. The lack of multidisciplinary cooperation in the planning and establishment of any hospital group program can lead to a negative outcome on both the intra- and extra-group level (Lonergan, 1982, p. 4; Lonergan, 1980). For groups with oncology patients, staff skepticism as to their feasibility and appropriateness can prove an obstacle to group process (Ringler et al., 1981).

Teamwork remains essential even after groups are established. This becomes especially obvious, and crucial for the single-session, when leadership is shared by members of two (or more) different professions (e.g., nursing and social work) that may have difference in perspective and group approach (Euster, 1979; Keith, 1980; Johnson and Stark, 1980).

Recruitment and Contract

The common experience of hospitalization itself, the *culture* of the hospital unit, and prior contact the group members may have had with staff can be viewed as part of the *pre-group* phase (Hartford,

1971, p. 67) of the single-session group. Recruitment becomes an opportunity for, what Schwartz (1968) called, *tuning in* (p. 334). Recruitment must also be conceptualized as the start of contracting and beginnings (Crawford, 1982). Thus while the patients are encouraged to attend, the worker's invitation must be clear, direct, and "no-nonsense" about what kind of participation is to be the goal (Bloom and Lynch, 1979; Ringler et al., 1981). Once each session formally begins, the contract must be restated. Despite the pressure of time, contracting remains critical (Shulman, 1979, p. 266).

Education as Structure

An educational component in groups serves the function of imparting of information, one of Yalom's (1975) eleven curative factors. Providing cancer patients with information about their illness and its treatment is seen as one of the most effective ways to help alleviate the sense of (and often real) loss of control that can accompany the diagnosis (Euster, 1979; Rickert and Koffmann, 1982).

Imparting of information, however, is only one step. Learning new information in any anxiety-laden area requires that emotional as well as intellectual needs be given attention (Lonergan, 1982; p. 235). The challenge in such groups, as Shulman (1979) states, is not only to present information but to elicit interaction to make it more meaningful.

An educational component can also help provide structural support in these single-session groups (Lonergan, 1982, p. 10). This component acts as an initial binding force. It provides an element of "formality," giving members a chance to "distance themselves" as they get used to each other's presence (*ibid.*, p. 239). This serves to increase the likelihood of both attendance and participation, since it helps the cancer patient over the initial difficulty in expressing and discussing his/her feelings (Barstow, 1982, p. 39), as well as increasing the level of anxiety the group members are able to tolerate.

Composition

The psychosocial problems of cancer patients can be transient and changeable. Weisman (Rickert and Koffman, 1982) has suggested the notion of *phases,* related to the clinical *stages* of cancer, to understand patients' concentration on different kinds of psychosocial problems at different times during their illnesses (p. 30). The problems vary as do the strategies employed to cope with them, for each person over time and among people at the same phase. This diversity of experience and lack of *synchrony* (Germain, 1976) has obvious implications for group treatment of cancer patients (Christ, 1982b; 1983). Needless to say, these implications are exaggerated in the case of a single-session.

The prescription generally given for group composition is enough homogeneity for commonality and enough heterogeneity for spontaneity (Lonergan, 1982, p. 12). For groups with a cancer population however, there is no agreement on this issue. Wood et al. (1978), for example, feel that patients at different stages of their cancer have trouble relating to one another. The groups they described were homogeneous for stage of disease but heterogenous for all other factors (except that all members were out-patients) (p. 558). Rickert and Koffmann (1982), however, recommend mixing patients (in- and out-) whose illnesses represent multiple disease sites (p. 40). They see the heterogeneous group as the most satisfactory format and the one best suited to both the realities of cancer and the logistics of medical care.

The crisis element inherent in hospitalization itself seems to afford in-patient groups the ability to tolerate more heterogeneity and dis-synchrony that would be normally expected (Lonergan, 1982, pp. 13-4). In oncology patient groups with their heightened sense of crisis, the commonality of the cancer diagnosis, often regardless of heterogeneous sites, can provide the potential for cohesion and serve as a *compensating variable* (Evans and Jarvis, 1980) for homogeneity.

Process and Cohesion in Transient Groups

No matter how it is defined, *cohesion* is usually described as a necessary, although perhaps not sufficient, condition for the improvement of group members. *Group cohesiveness* is yet another one of Yalom's (1975) curative factors. Yalom has also referred to a stable membership as the *sine qua non* of successful group therapy (Evans and Jarvis, 1980, p. 405).

Bailis et al. (1978), however, propose that there is a cohesion that exists even in open groups despite the constant turnover in membership. These authors use the term *legacy* to describe the transmission of group norms and values from one group *generation* to another which, despite its transiency, seems to stabilize the group.

Golland (1972) and Hoch (1955) agree that open-endedness and/or time-limited involvement are not mutually exclusive for the development of either group norms or phases. Despite time limits and transiency, in both leader- and membership, Johnson and Stark (1980) have noted a sense of "intimacy" reached by many groups for cancer patients. Important when considering the single-session group is the implication here that the level of group structure (e.g., beginning) does not necessarily determine that of process.

Phases

It is generally acknowledged that there are phases through which a group passes—a developmental sequence—and that the tasks of both leaders and members vary depending on the *age* of the group (Garland et al., 1973). Beginnings, middles, and ends (and the accompanying dynamic stances between members and leaders) also exist for short-term groups, although in a condensed manner (Northen, 1969). This is equally true for each individual session of any group that meets over a period of time, be it short- or long-term (Shulman, 1979).

For the single-session group, "the same logic and the same necessities of work make the terms of the analysis equally applicable" (Schwartz and Zalba, 1971, p. 13). Problem-solving groups that meet for one session proceed through a predictable sequence (Bales, 1970), and groups meeting for only a few hours follow a very similar phasic course to those that run for a period of a year (Shalinsky, 1981, p. 8).

Shulman (1979) maintains that each single-session "meeting" be viewed as a *small group*, even though he tends to see the single-session as larger and more for the purposes of providing information and education than emotional support and interaction (p. 266). Tuning in, contracting, work, and termination phases all are encompassed in one session. "The one-session group," writes Schwartz (1968), "(gives) us the opportunity to study the working construct of beginning, middle, and end as it applie(s) in the space of a single meeting" (p. 356).

Casper (1981) introduces the concept of *concurrent* phases to the more traditional linear and spiral models. He suggests that all stages exist, to some degree, in every group at all times. Within a short-term group and each individual session within its time frame, there is a beginning, climax, end, and *episodes* (*ibid.*, p. 4). For the single-session group, this notion is very helpful in conceptualizing the dis-synchrony that often exists between process and structure, i.e., that the two are "out of phase," or at different levels of phasic development.

Group Evolution

A framework for conceptualizing the single-session group requires that one be attuned to its time limits and the structural ramifications of these limits. Lang's (1972) formulation distinguishes three orders of groups and offers an additional dynamic dimension to the ideas presented above.

The three group orders (*allonomous, allon-autonomous* or transitional, and *autonomous*) fall along a continuum of increasing structural complexity and decreasing worker activity. On one end is the characteristic worker-directed functioning of the allonomous group form. On the other is the group-as-a-whole functioning of the autonomous form, with the worker assuming a less active role (Lang, 1972, p. 85).

Shalinsky (1981) uses this model to analyze the single-session group and concludes that the transition described above is possible even within the lifespan of one individual meeting. The level of group structure and process attained, however, depends to a large extent on the worker's ability to assume a central and active role (p. 17). As suggested earlier, a single-session may at times represent a group of a different order but not basically a different kind.

Role of the Leader(s)

Working with the single-session takes a leader who is skilled and comfortable with groups and has the flexibility of skills needed for all short-term work (Lonergan, 1982; Cory, 1982; Wolberg, 1965; Hoch, 1965; Wolf, 1965). "Single-session groups require specialized skills on the part of the leader—tuning in to the group members' needs, contracting, getting into the work, and termination—all in one or two hours" (Poynter-Berg and Weiner, 1979, p. 37). The worker must set proper conditions which enable group members to work effectively (Shulman, 1979, pp. 267-68). For the cancer patient, these conditions include the creation of a safe group environment (Ringler et al., 1981).

Lang's (1972) model implies that all group workers must be able to shift roles and activities quickly and flexibly in order to encourage group development. Along her continuum, the role of the worker evolves from a central (*surrogate*) to peripheral (*facilitating*) locus. In the middle lies the *significant constituent*, the worker in the transitional group, who must pivot between being a surrogate and facilitator, keeping up with member readiness to deal autonomously (pp. 85-6). Such a sensitivity to both limitations and potential is that which is required of the single-session worker.

In crisis groups, the active role of the worker is said to serve as a model to the members (Germain, 1976; Strickler and Allgeyer, 1967; Allgeyer, 1973; Smith, 1979). Important for the single-session worker as well is the attitude that recognizes the need to make the most of limited time and encourages group members to do the same (Shalinsky, 1981, p. 16).

Leader(s') Goals and Expectations

Contract, goals, and worker expectations in single-session groups, as in crisis and all short-term work, must be limited, realistic and geared to the patients' needs (Lonergan, 1982). As Casper (1981) recommends, "never start anything you can't finish" (p. 3).

Shalinsky (1981) suggests that it is perhaps wise to expect interpersonal relationships in these groups to be at a more superficial level than in longer-term groups (p. 14). His comment serves as a reminder of the necessity for tailored purposes and limited objectives.

But Wolf (1965) and Yalom and Greaves (1977) leave the worker with a caveat—that it is often s/he who is responsible for superficiality in group interaction. Reservations may stem more from the fact that needs of the leaders are not being met than those of the patients cannot be met (Lonergan, 1982, p. 11). With oncology patients, countertransferential issues for the leaders can prove an obstacle to group development (Ringler et al., 1981).

With regard to oncology groups, there is the issue of the appropriateness, especially on such a short-term basis, of encouraging members to confront painful and often existential issues. Rickert and Koffmann (1982) see the worker's role to prevent discussion from becoming too *concrete*, i.e., obsessed with the medical aspects of cancer to the exclusion of its psychosocial ones. Workers should feel comfortable in encouraging the exploration of anxiety-producing material (*ibid.*, p. 40).

The above literature review supports the view that single-session groups for cancer patients are both appropriate and feasible. Perhaps this is best summarized by the following quote (Ringler et al., 1981):

> ...(H)aving cancer is a crisis situation that brings out people's strengths and also acts as a prod, making them willing and able to use a less than ideal situation—group meetings that they attend only once or twice—to expose their difficulties and to gain support and new alternatives for handling them. (p. 342)

The Single-Session Group: Process and Approach

Group Formation

The group on Memorial Hospital's surgical gynecology floor is offered to the women as a mode of providing information and mutual support to help them cope with their losses—loss of identity, loss of control, loss of social support, and the loss of the perception of unending time (Euster, 1979; Rickert and Koffmann, 1982).

Because of its time-limited nature, the suggested intent for the single-session group is to provide supportive rather than analytic intervention. Using Slavson's (1979) framework, these groups can be said to straddle the line between a *guidance* and *counselling* group. The goal can thus be seen as *symptom relief* for the cancer patient, as well as increased awareness and improvement of reality testing and other skills.

The group's purpose is to facilitate the learning of information and the utilization of this in an adaptive rather than defensive intellectualized way. The worker's aim is to provide an environment where the patients can feel comfortable airing concerns and, perhaps, even existential issues. The worker's goal becomes one of encouraging the exploration of anxiety while maintaining the responsibility for providing conditions that will help to contain it.

All women hospitalized on the gynecological unit are invited to attend, all who have been admitted for work-up and/or treatment of gynecological conditions be they malignant or benign. Some who attend the group are still awaiting diagnostic test results; others are scheduled for their initial surgery; yet others have been readmitted for treatment of recurrent disease by radio- and/or chemotherapy. A few have just learned their disease is benign.

The size of the convened group tends to vary from 3-5 to 8-10; the most workable number being 5-7. The resulting membership for any one of these single-session groups is both homogeneous (e.g., sex, patient status, cancer diagnosis, treatments) and heterogeneous (e.g., site of gynecological disease, particular cancer type, stage of disease).

Recruitment is the time for tuning in and for initiation of contracting between workers and potential group members. If it is successful, members will enter the group understanding the contract, purpose, and their expected role.

Worker confidence and competence, as well as ambivalence, is reflected in recruitment style. The gynecology group, for example, is presented as a place for discussion where patients can talk about their concerns, ask questions about procedures, etc. Its volunteer and participatory nature is stressed but its *true* intent must also be communicated. That is, that while the nurse and/or social worker will impart information and answer concrete questions, the focus is on mutual support and the exploration of more psychosocial issues. This recruitment invitation then becomes the basis for contracting once the group is convened.

At the beginning of each single-session, the worker must be prepared to make a very clear and concise statement on the purpose and goals of the group, and be willing to invite comment and offer clarification as quickly as possible. Contracting is a continuation of the process initiated during recruitment. It remains essential in these groups despite the pressure of time, or perhaps because of the focus necessitated by it. A technique suggested is to ask each group member how the group can be useful to him/her that day and emphasize the one-time-only quality of the group (MSKCC, 1983, B).

The necessity for such a clear statement has implications for the worker as well. Without clarification, there can be an inability to distinguish problems that are due to ambiguity in contract from those that arise out of group process or worker interventions (or lack of them).

With self-awareness, a worker's hesitation about a more *confrontational* style may have to be acknowledged as "right now I feel unable, or judge it to be unwise" rather than "I have no right" when it comes to encouraging exploration of more anxiety-producing themes. Contract thus helps to clarify for the worker issues of feasibility, appropriateness, confidence, competence, and/or countertransference. The necessity for such a distinction exists in any group. But it is of paramount importance both in a single session group and with a cancer population.

Group Processes

During recruitment for the gynecology group, the educational component (including a nurse as co-leader) helps to *sell* the group. Indeed, the social worker who initially established the group concluded that the use of the word *meeting* rather than *group* resulted in a much more favorable recruitment response (MSKCC, 1983, C). Patients who are reluctant to attend seem to feel less threatened that they will be "forced" to speak knowing there will be an objective focus provided by the nurse. The educational piece provides the distance often needed in beginnings and makes the group seem a safer space. Oftentimes it is those women who are initially the most reluctant to attend who become the most active participants.

Since each of these groups begins afresh one might say that these single-sessions are constantly starting over. But a certain degree of commonality already does exist among the women recruited for the gynecology group. The shared experience of hospitalization, surgery, and/or the diagnosis of cancer seems to create some sense of intimacy and helps provide the basis, or potential, for rapport among group participants.

Is there also a *legacy* that exists for the single-session? Are there some compensating variables for cohesion and continuity?

In these one-shot affairs the leaders can be said to be the *carriers of the flame.* They provide the continuity which is supplied by the compensating factor of meeting frequency in some open-ended groups. An active leadership role helps to hasten group process. Hospital routine, staff support, shared recruitment, and previous (or subsequent) member contact with group leaders also contribute to a sense of ongoingness.

Members themselves also come with their various experiences, skills, and capacities gained in other groups and events. They too bring a picture of what each particular single-session will be all about and thus become a part of its past as well as its future (Shalinsky, 1981). Each one-shot is a *generation* unto itself.

With a 1-1/2-hour meeting, it has been suggested (Shalinsky, 1981) that a group can be beyond the *beginning* and *exploring* stages by the end of 30 minutes and well into the phase of *group functioning.* One then has only 15 minutes for the review, feedback, and anticipation of *termination* (p. 14). A worker must be able to shift roles and activities quickly and flexibly, like the significant constituent of Lang's (1972) transitional group form.

The final form that exists at the end of any single-session will, of course, very much depend on the *functioning* of the members. If the women attending the gynecology group, for instance, have attended the same or similar group during previous hospitalizations, a transitional or autonomous group might develop with the worker's active encouragement. But if no member has ever been in a group before, the worker should not take it as a sign of "defeat" if the level of interaction exhibits more that of a guidance group or allonomous form (Shalinsky, 1981, p. 15). Indeed, such a group form might be the most appropriate for that particular collection of individuals.

Role of the Leader(s)

Time is so limited in these groups that the leader(s) have to intervene so as to speed up the process whereby the group members can develop a rapport and sense of commonality in purpose and need. Leaders need to encourage all to participate early on, clearly delineate raised themes (manifest and/or latent), and allow sufficient time for an ending. Closure is always crucial in the single-session but this need becomes intensified when working with a cancer population.

The active leadership style required serves as a role model for the level of group interaction. But the worker must exercise judgement to achieve for each single-session the proper balance between *structure* and *independence*. Ringler et al. (1981) speak of the need to achieve a balance between *intrusiveness* and *abandonment* (p. 342). Patients need to be reassured of their ability to tolerate anxiety and encouraged to be assertive in investigating the details of their illness and planned treatment. Although the worker's role remains a central one, the goal is to facilitate and to provide for the group neither too much nor too little in terms of structure and direction. A leader who is unnecessarily directive promotes infantalization, a potential for which already exists in the *culture of patienthood* (*ibid.*, p. 340) and which must be counteracted if an individual is to succeed in the task of coping with his/her cancer.

Regardless of the particular setting, the one-shot deal is inherently *out of synch*. Even at its ending group process seems to constantly demand a leadership style that is explicitly active and sometimes

directive, one that is usually thought appropriate to only the beginning phase. In a sense, such *dis-synchrony* becomes the motivating
force behind a successful single-session group.

Conclusion

> In my beginning is my end . . . So here I am . . . and every
> attempt is a wholly new start, a raid on the inarticulate . . .
> And so each venture is a new beginning . . . And what there is
> to conquer has already been discovered once or twice, or sev-
> eral times . . . and (also) under conditions that seem unpro-
> pitious . . . For us there is only the trying. The rest is not our
> business. In my end is my beginning. (T.S. Eliot, 1962)

Although these single-session groups are widely used in hospital
settings, there remains an ambivalence about their feasibility, effectiveness, and appropriateness, even amongst some leaders themselves. These sixty minute encounters can appear deceptively simple
from the outside. They need to become more of a focus for in-
vestigation which will outline suggestions for differential approaches to recruitment and intervention, as well as particular concerns for
specialized settings.

A *good enough* single-session group depends on planning, purpose, and structure. For these components to be effective, however,
depends largely on the worker. S/he must be able to assure and take
responsibility for a central role in group process and feel comfortable and confident that such a role is both appropriate and
necessary. But s/he must also remain sensitive and respond flexibly
to each individual group's need for structure. There is room for
variation in development among single-session groups. Not all start
out or finish at the same level of process. Worker flexibility and
confidence, reflected from the outset in the recruitment approach,
can be a motivating force for members. Such an attitude makes conditions seem far less "unpropitious."

But while one must be optimistic and hopeful, one must also face
and accept reality. Living with uncertainty and potential time limits
must become the *modus vivendi* of the cancer patient. So too the
leaders of these one-shot deals need to be confronted with the ac-
tualities of *partipotence* (Wolf, 1965, p. 247) inherent in all short-
term work. Time is limited, goals must be limited, and standards for
evaluation need to be determined by limited objectives. To seek

perfection is always unwise. For the single-session group leader it becomes impossible. Besides, to what perfect model would one aspire?

"For us there is only the trying . . ." To say "(t)he rest is not our business" is not to assume or admit failure. Rather, it is a recognition of both the potentiality and limits of the single-session group. These groups are not panaceas. What they do is to help provide information and/or emotional support. Working with a cancer population is a constant testimony to these people's strengths and capabilities. But their adaptive tasks remain difficult nonetheless. In the final analysis, it is the individual member him/herself who must incorporate the group experience. Each "possesses the only real and lasting means to his(/her) own ends" (Schwartz, 1961, p. 153).

But the leaders of single-session groups need to constantly (re)examine whether they themselves, through particular style or technique or lack of contract, are inadvertently providing *obstacles to the search for common ground.* The time constraints serve only to exaggerate a need that actually exists for leaders of all groups, be they short- or long-term.

There exists a certain parallel process between the single-session worker and this author who has contracted with her reader to convey a sense of the group in this *one-shot* paper. The goals of both are similar—to clearly present purpose, establish organizing structure, maintain focus, and gauge content and depth according to the limits of space and time. Ideally for both, if such goals are achieved the potentiality of their limits will have been realized.

"In (this) end is (a) beginning"—hopefully, a beginning handbook for the single-session worker.

REFERENCES

Allgeyer, J. (1973). Using groups in a crisis-oriented out-patient setting. *International Journal of Group Psychotherapy, 23,* 217-22.

Bales, R.F. (1970). A set of categories for the analysis of small group interaction, in D.P. Forcese and S. Richer (Eds.), *Stages of Social Research. Contemporary Perspectives* (pp. 216-24). Englewood Cliffs: Prentice-Hall.

Bailis, S.S., Lambert, S.R., & Bernstein, S.B. (1978). The legacy of the group: a study of a group therapy with a transient membership. *Social Work in Health Care, 3*(4), 405-18.

Barstow, L.F. (1982). Working with cancer patients in radiation therapy. *Health and Social Work, 7*(1), 35-40.

Bloom, N.D., & Lynch, J.G. (1979). Group work in a hospital waiting room. *Health and Social Work, 4*(3), 48-63.

Casper, M. (1981). The short-term group: a special case in social work. Paper presented at the Third Annual Symposium on the Advancement of Social Work with Groups, Hartford, Conn., October. In M. Goroff (Ed.), *Reaping from the field—from practice to principle: Proceedings three* (pp. 733-756). Hebron, CT: Practitioners Press.

Christ, G. (1982a). Use of groups in psychosocial care of cancer patients. In J.C. Holland (Ed.), *Current Concepts in Psychosocial Oncology: Effects of Cancer and its Treatment on Patient, Family and Staff.* Syllabus of the Postgraduate Course. Memorial Sloan-Kettering Cancer Center, October.

Christ, G. (1982b). "Dis-synchrony" of coping among children with cancer, their families, and the treating staff. In A.E. Christ and K. Flomenhaft (Eds.), *Family Theory and Family Therapy in Pediatric Illness* (pp. 85-95). New York: Plenum Press.

Christ, G. (1983). A psychosocial assessment framework for cancer patients and their families. *Health and Social Work, 8*(1), 57-64.

Cory, T.L. (1982). Techniques for accelerating awareness in short-term group psychotherapy. *Small Group Behavior, 13*(2), 259-63.

Crawford, J. (1982). Improving recruitment for family groups in an acute-care hospital. Paper submitted for Integrative Seminar, Hunter College School of Social Work, Spring.

Dinerman, M., Schlesinger, E.G., & Wood, K.M. (1980). Social work roles in health care: an educational framework. *Health and Social Work, 5*(4), 13-20.

Eliot, T.S. (1962). "East Coker," from "Four Quartets." In *The Complete Poems and Plays* (pp. 123-29). New York: Harcourt, Brace and World, Inc.

Euster, S. (1979). Rehabilitation after mastectomy: the group process. *Social Work in Health Care, 4*(3), 251-263.

Evans, N.J., & Jarvis, P.A. (1980). Group cohesion. A review and reevaluation. *Small Group Behavior, 11*(4), 359-70.

Falck, H.S. (1978). Social work in health settings. *Social Work in Health Care, 3*(4), 395-403.

Frankl, V.E. (1973). *Man's Search for Meaning.* New York: Pocket Books.

Garland, J.A., Jones, H.E., & Kolodny, R. (1973). A model for stages of development in social work groups. In S. Bernstein (Ed.), *Explorations in Group Work: Essays in Theory and Practice* (pp. 12-53). Boston: Boston University School of Social Work.

Germain, C.B. (1976). Time: an ecological variable in social work practice. *Social Casework, 57*(7), 419-26.

Golland, J.H. (1972). A "hello" and "goodbye" group. *International Journal of Psychotherapy, 22*(2), 248-61.

Hartford, M.E. (1971). *Groups in Social Work.* New York: Columbia University Press.

Hoch, P. H. (1965). Short-term versus long-term therapy. In L.R. Wolberg (Ed.), *Short-Term Psychotherapy* (p. 61). New York: Grune and Stratton.

Hoch, E.L., & Kaufer, G. (1955). A process analysis of "transient" therapy groups. *International Journal of Group Psychotherapy, 5,* 415-21.

Johnson, E.M., & Stark, D.W. (1980). A group program for cancer patients and their family members in an acute care teaching hospital. *Social Work in Health Care, 5*(4), 335-49.

Keith, C. (1980). Discussion group for posthysterectomy patients. *Health and Social Work, 5*(1), 59-63.

Konopka, G. (1963). *Social Group Work: A Helping Process.* Englewood Cliffs: Prentice-Hall.

Lang, N. (1972). A broad-range model of practice in the social work group. *Social Service Review, 46,* 76-89.

Lonergan, E.C. (1980). Humanizing the hospital experience: report of a group program for medical patients. *Health and Social Work, 5*(4), 53-63.

Lonergan, E.C. (1982). *Group Intervention. How to Begin and Maintain Groups in Medical and Psychiatric Settings.* New York: Jason Aronson.

MSKCC (1983). Personal communication with four social workers at Memorial Hospital: (A) Mary Wall, CSW; (B) Lois Weinstein, CSW; (C) Martha Atchley, CSW; (D) Mary Ellen Bowles, MS, CSW.

Northen, H. (1969). *Social Work with Groups.* New York: Columbia University Press.

Poynter-Berg, D., & Weiner, H. (1979). *Workshop Summaries. Social Work with Groups in Maternal and Child Health.* New York: Columbia University and Roosevelt Hospital.

Rickert, M.L., & Koffmann, A. (1982). The Use of Groups with Cancer Patients. In M. Seligman (Ed.), *Group Psychotherapy and Counseling with Special Populations* (pp. 27-41). Baltimore: University Park Press.

Ringler, K.E. et al. (1981). Technical advances in leading a cancer patient group. *International Journal of Psychotherapy, 31*(3), 329-43.

Robinovitch, A.E., & Ransohoff, M.E. (1981). Group work in general hospitals. Crisis intervention and politics. *Social Work with Groups, 4*(3/4), 59-66.

Schwartz, M.D. (1975). Situation/transition groups: a conceptualization and review. *American Journal of Orthopsychiatry, 45*(5), 744-55.

Schwartz, W. (1961). The social worker in the group. *Social Welfare Forum,* 1961, 146-71.

Schwartz, W. (1968). Group work in public welfare. *Public Welfare, 26*(4), 322-70.

Schwartz, W. & Zalba, S. (Eds.), (1971). *The Practice of of Group Work.* New York: Columbia University Press.

Shalinsky, W. (1981). One session meetings: aggregate or group? Paper presented at the Third Annual symposium on the Advancement of Social Work with Groups, Hartford, Conn., October.

Shulman, L. (1979). *The Skills of Helping Individuals and Groups.* Itasca, Ill.: F.E. Peacock.

Slavson, S.R. (1979). When is a therapy group not a therapy group? In *Dynamics of Group Psychotherapy* (pp. 201-221). New York: Jason Aronson, pp. 201-221.

Smith, L.L. (1979). Crisis intervention in practice. *Social Casework, 60*(2), 81-88.

Spiegel, D., & Yalom, I.D. (1978). A support group for dying patients. *International Journal of Group Psychotherapy, 28*(2), 233-45.

Strickler, M. & Allgeyer, J. (1967). The crisis group: a new application of crisis theory. *Social Work, 12,* 28-32.

Trillin, A.S. (1981). Of dragons and garden peas. A cancer patient talks to doctors. *New England Journal of Medicine, 304*(12), 699-701.

Weiner, H.J. (1959). The hospital, the ward, and the patient as clients: use of the group method. *Social Work, 4*(4), 57-64.

Wolberg, L.R. (1965). The technic of short-term psychotherapy. In L.R. Wolberg (Ed.), *Short-Term Psychotherapy* (pp. 127-95). New York: Grune and Stratton.

Wolf, A. (1965). Short-term group psychotherapy. In L.R. Wolberg (Ed.), *ibid.,* 219-50.

Wood, P.E. et al. (1978). Group counselling for cancer patients in a community hospital. *Psychosomatic Medicine, 19*(9), 555-58.

Yalom, I.D. (1979). *The Theory and Practice of Group Psychotherapy.* Second Edition. New York: Basic Books.

Yalom, I.D., & Greaves, C. (1977). Group therapy with the terminally ill. *American Journal of Psychiatry, 134*(4), 396-400.

Children's Single-Session Briefings: Group Work with Military Families Experiencing Parents' Deployment

Jane A. Waldron
Ronaele R. Whittington
Steve Jensen

ABSTRACT. Forced separation of a parent from the family because of military service creates a crisis for all family members. A series of children's single-session briefings involved talking with parents and children in a large group, talking with children in small groups while their parents observed and then large group discussion with parents. The children were encouraged to express feelings related to separation and parents were assisted in developing strategies for coping with the family changes resulting from the deployments. The children's briefings were organized pre- , mid- and post-deployment and utilized lecture, slides, and coloring books. The groups were led by two clinical social workers and a chaplain.

Forced separation of a parent from the family because of military service creates a crisis for all family members (Bonovich, 1967). Military families routinely experience separation of a parent, most often the father, due to his non-accompanied military tours ranging from periods of weeks to a year. Father absence has been correlated with the high incidence of behavioral disorders in children of military families (Yeatman, 1981; Lagrone, 1978; Bloom, 1969; Dickerson and Arthur, 1965). Intrapsychic conflicts in wives and children of military fathers absent from home have been reported by

Jane A. Waldron, PhD, is Associate Professor of Psychiatry, John A. Burns School of Medicine, Honolulu, Hawaii, and also the Director of the Children's Divorce Clinic at Kapiolani-Children's Medical Center, Honolulu, Hawaii. Address correspondence to Dr. Waldron at Kapiolani-Children's Medical Center, Child Guidance Center, 1319 Punahou Street, Honolulu, Hawaii 96826. Ronaele R. Whittington, DSW is a social worker in private practice in Kailua, Hawaii. Steve Jensen, Chaplain, U. S. Navy, is currently stationed at the Marine Corps Air Station, Kaneohe Bay, Hawaii.

many authors (Cretekos, 1971; Bey and Lange, 1974; Gonzalez, 1970; Pearlman, 1970; Cove, Fagen, and Barker, 1969; Lester, 1977). Separations of military fathers from their children have been found to substantially alter the development of the children's conscience formation and their ability to relate to others (Crumley and Blumenthal, 1973; Biller, 1973). In addition, the return of the absent parent has been noted to produce stress on spouse and child (Lagrone, 1978; Butterworth, 1979; den Dulk and Hunter, 1981). Many authors cite the need for the development of interventions to assist military families in coping with the enforced parental absence (Bonovich, 1967, Lagrone, 1978, Yeatman, 1981).

The military is a huge organization and, like other bureaucracies, it is characterized by a strong authoritative hierarchy. Individuality is discouraged; compliance to the rules and goals of the organization is stressed; confrontation is actively discouraged and families are treated as necessary but often troublesome additions to the system. Moreover, the very nature and diversity of family living patterns are changing, leaving greater numbers of factors to be considered in dealing with families (Bowen, 1981). The military strives to bind its members tightly in order to carry out its objectives of national defense. Outside relationships, specifically families, are secondary to those objectives. The family's value and rights exist only through the military parent. In such a setting, family relationships are at risk for problems. Some investigators have found that the absence of fathers from the family increases the rate of emotional disturbance, violence and incest within these families (Bobrowsky, 1982; Groth, Hobson, and Gary, 1982; Kovalesky-McLaine, 1982).

Some authors have cited enforced separation of a parent the most severe stress of a military family (Lagrone, 1978). In the most common situation, father absence, the mother is forced to take over responsibilities of both parents. This produces an increase in mothers' independence, a shift in roles and routines, and commonly generates depression, anxiety and anger in military spouses. Once a family has adapted to the changes in its functioning required by fathers' absence, reintegration of the absent parent is necessary. This can be as stressful as the original adjustment. Under the stress of repeated and extended separations, submarine wives experience symptoms of headaches, back aches, occasional insomnia, temporary loss of muscle power, periodic depression, short temper, minor weight changes, edginess and tension. In one study, seventeen per cent experienced excessive anxiety symptoms—tightness in the throat, extended shortness of breath, repeated deep sighing, tightness in the chest, problem with elimination, and extended periods of tearfulness. Changes in these symptoms were likened to stages of grief—shock, denial, anger, depression, loneliness, aggression, hostility, despair and reintegration (Bermudes, 1973).

The military has long been criticized for its anti-family stance which appears to separate families with little consideration of the impact on the family unit. Within the past five years, however, there has been some effort to assist families in coping with deployments (Coigney, 1981; den Dulk and Hunter, 1981; Ebbert, 1980; Family Program Support Division, Department of the Navy, 1981; Girard, 1982; Lexier, 1981; Parry and Parkenson, 1981)

History

The model to be presented in this paper is one that was based on efforts that began in January 1981 at the Naval Submarine base in New London, Conn. An ombudswoman for the USS Andrew Jackson arranged for a predeployment briefing for the children of the submarine's crew. Two social workers participated in that session working with the children and the parents separately in two twenty-minute long groups. Leaders for the group included the commanding officer, executive officer and other ship's personnel. The children received an explanation of what their fathers did on the ship, the importance of their jobs and the reasons for the deployments. Feelings of patriotism and pride were stressed. A slide show of the last patrol, refreshments and gifts, which included note pads for the children to write to their dads, were included in the experience.

Following that briefing, the first to our knowledge, a children's coloring book was created which was intended to remind the children of the material covered during the briefing. At this point the base social worker, unit chaplain and the Commodore's wife, who was also a social worker, became part of the team developing the model of children's briefings. This group had a distinct advantage in the clear support it received from the naval command structure. Important concepts developed by that creative group included (1) the importance of children understanding what deployments are about, (2) the importance of children expressing feelings related to deployments, (3) the need to assist parents in developing ways to keep dad in the family during his absence, (4) the need to encourage continued communication between separated parents and their children, (5) the need to assist families in developing strategies for coping with the family changes resulting from the deployment. The family was encouraged to continue in dad's absence and the family was given help in dealing with the various transitions.

In 1982, the chaplain who had been involved in the New London children's briefings was transferred to the Marine Corps Air Station at Kaneohe Bay, Hawaii. He set out to institute children's briefings for the families of this base and was able to secure funds to support the involvement of two child-oriented clinical social workers to assist in the development of children's briefings in Hawaii. The new program utilized some of the materials developed in the previous program. Coloring books were redrawn by the Marines Graphic Arts to depict Marines on both ships and planes. The model developed in Hawaii relied heavily on children's groups as a means to reach children and to teach parents how to assist their children through this crisis. Parents were encouraged to observe the children's groups in order to better acquaint them with their children's emotions and to offer models of how to handle them appropriately. Sessions were called Children's Briefings in keeping with military jargon and were held with families at a variety of points in the deployment process. Some briefings were held just prior to the parent's leaving, within two weeks after deployment, midway in the deployment and just prior to the father's return. The differences in attitude of the various officers in command of the deployed groups heavily influenced when or whether a Children's Briefing was held.

Format

The Briefings were organized in most cases by the ombudsperson working closely with the chaplain's office. The meetings were scheduled at a variety of times, some on Sunday afternoons and some during the week, in the early evening. Meeting place varied, i.e., Enlisted Men's Club, Officers' Club, Base Chapel, Family Services Center. The sessions lasted one and a half hours and were co-led by the chaplain and the two social workers. Attention to logistics and facilities was very important. Noise from nearby competing activities, poor lighting or late starts during evening meetings decreased the effectiveness of the briefings.

Meetings began with the parents and their children in one group. A short statement was made about the purpose of the meeting and the common stress that the families experience when fathers are away for long periods of time. The coloring book for children, which depicted military families experiencing a father's deployment, was distributed. Slides made from the coloring book were then shown and used as a basis for discussion with the parents and children about some of the concrete issues which related to deployments. The pictures depicted Marines in various jobs, Marines preparing for departure, ships and planes on maneuvers, families in various activities without dad present and finally the homecoming and reuniting of fathers and their families. Also distributed was a copy of a pamphlet written by students at the base elementary school about what it's like to have dad gone on deployment. The main points of this pamphlet, which focused on children's reactions and feelings, were summarized. Discussion of this handout was intended to give the children permission to discuss a range of feelings related to dad's absence.

Next, children five years old and over were invited to join a small group of ten to fifteen children to talk about their experiences. The groups were led by the social workers. Children were asked to sit in a semi-circle, often on the floor, if the facilities were clean and carpeted. Parents were encouraged to sit on the outside of the group and observe. Group discussion lasted approximately thirty minutes.

Issues for children were somewhat different depending on the families' positions in the deployment process. Families who had not yet experienced the parent leaving tended to be in a denial stage where activity predominated and little discussion of the departure was occurring. Feelings about the upcoming separation were painful for all and some parents expressed apprehension about attending briefings. Focus during these briefings was on the changes that the family would be facing, feelings which were commonly evoked by those changes, and ways to cope with the changes. Parents' ability to deny feelings was most often stronger than that of their children. In the small group discussions the children readily talked of their sadness, worries and anger about dad going away.

All groups focused first on concrete issues like when dad was leaving, where he was going, how long he would be gone, what he would be doing and why he was going. Some children had no information and others were well-informed. Discussion then moved into changes that would occur as a result of dad's absence and what that might feel like. Often children in the groups had already experienced deployments and could share their experiences. Changes involved less people to do the work of the family, chores being redistributed and there being only one adult to handle discipline and decision making. This latter issue was sometimes seen as good and sometimes seen as bad by the children.

Many children were frank, articulate and verbal about their sadness, anger, fears and sometimes relief at having dad gone. The discussions got quickly into how their mothers acted differently in that they were often sad and irritable and how, at first especially, it was very painful to have dad gone. Children shared the things they did which made them feel better. These ranged from keeping busy and not thinking about dad, to cuddling up with mom and crying, to writing to dad, to going to the beach or to McDonald's and having fun. The anger and the worries expressed by the children seemed to be of most surprise to parents since these were feelings least often discussed at home. Ways of keeping dad part of the family during his absence were discussed, i.e., putting a picture of dad in the child's room, taking lots of pictures of family activities before dad left.

Following the children's groups the parents and children reassembled into one group and the leaders reviewed the pertinent feelings, concerns and issues which arose in the groups, and talked about ways parents could assist children in dealing with common stresses. A discussion period with parents and children together allowed for focus on more individualized concerns. A list of coping strategies and the local resources for help with child-related problems was discussed with the group. The session ended with refreshments and families were encouraged to socialize with each other. The presence of food of some kind was felt to be important in creating a nurturant, friendly atmosphere for these families experiencing stress.

Group Dynamics

From a group dynamics standpoint, these children's groups, offered within the context of a highly-structured, homogeneous military organization, and focusing on a common experience, are different from the usual therapeutic groups offered to children in the general community. Group cohesion formed quickly due to the fact that all of the families already belong to a larger group, the military. Most of the children live in the same community, go to the same schools and often socialize with each other. To some extent a group culture already exists, a common military language or jargon is in use and all of the children have familiarity with military lifestyle. A group bond, enhanced by these factors, strengthens the impact of the limited group experience.

'Old timers' or children who have experienced previous deployments are identified early in the group meeting and encouraged to relate their experiences. This stresses the commonality of the experience and gives the group members a sense that the experience can be mastered. Common norms and values are clearly present in the groups as the children talk about the importance of their fathers' jobs and the 'good' things the dads are doing to 'defend the country.'

What becomes clear very quickly is that, despite the noble and patriotic reasons for dads absence, the children have strong negative and ambivalent feelings about the absence. The fact that these feelings are shared leads rapidly to the expression of strong negative feelings in an atmosphere that feels safe and accepting. The groups often include siblings, school mates and friends who already feel comfortable with one another. Sharing begins easily. Older children often talk about their own feelings by describing their observations of their younger sibling's reactions.

Social Worker's Role

The role of the social worker is clearly one of facilitating the expression of feelings, identifying the more verbal, articulate children who can share information and feelings, and stimulating the participation of other children. Occasionally a child is made uncomfortable by the discussion and becomes restless or wanders away from the group. Others may have tears in their eyes and find the discussion painful. At these times, the group leaders must use clinical judgment in deciding how much stress an individual or the group can tolerate. A focus on successful coping strategies and upon helping oneself feel better, can relieve excessive tension. Turning the discussion to homecoming and the reuniting of the absent parent with the family reminds the children that the separation is limited in duration and that, although it is painful, it will end. The notion that while the family undergoes many changes with deployment, it still remains a family, is important for supporting a sense of security in the children.

While leading the groups, the social worker must be careful to involve children of varying ages in order to keep all the children interested. Younger children respond well to 'what' questions, i.e., What does dad's ship look like?; What are your chores while dad is away? This type of question allows younger children to participate in the discussion successfully. 'Why' questions, or feeling oriented questions can be directed at older children whose cognitive development is further along. In general, the discussion respects the developmental differences among the children and is kept simple and fast moving to keep the participation and interest high.

Future Directions

The authors are currently developing a game for use during the briefings to facilitate the process described above. A game format is used. Children draw cards from a deck and are asked to respond to the question or directions on the card. Typical deployment-related issues are covered by the questions and directions, i.e., Show how your mom acts when she is missing your dad; Tell one feeling a girl experienced the day her dad left on float; What extra chore did the ten year old boy have to do while his dad was away on deployment; Name one thing that children can do when they feel sad. This game may be used by families to facilitate discussion of deployment issues or by sensitive volunteers in working with families facing deployments. The advantage of a game format is that it allows children to deal with feelings at a distance. The group format enables children who cannot deal with their own feelings to hear how other children feel and cope.

The authors feel that the past two years' efforts in conducting deployment-related children's groups have been effective in assisting families to cope with the stress of fathers' absence. In order to support the expansion of child-oriented mental health services in military settings, further research about the specific impact of such interventions is needed. The climate is ripe for the development of family-oriented strategies as the military has become more cognizant of the importance of insuring the mental health of its active duty personnel by supporting the mental health of the military family.

REFERENCES

Bermudes, R.W. (1973). A ministry to the repeatedly grief stricken. *The Journal of Pastoral Care, 27,* 218-227.

Bey, D.R., & Lange, J. (1974). Wailing wives, women under stress. *American Journal of Psychiatry, 131,* 283-286.

Biller, H.B. (1973). *Father, Child and Sex Role.* Lexington, Mass.: D.C. Heath and Co.

Bloom, W. (1969). The chap clinic revisited. Presented at the 16th annual conference of Air Force Behavioral Scientists, Brooks Air Force Base, Texas. *January.*

Bobrowsky, S. (1982). The silent cry: child abuse in the military. *Ladycom, 9,* 1982.

Bonovich, R.C. (1967). The family crisis of enforced separation. Presented at the 14th annual conference of Air Force Behavioral Scientists, Brooks Air Force Base, Texas. *January.*

Bowen, G.L. (1981). Family patterns of U.S. military personnel. N.A.S.W. Professional Symposium, Philadelphia, Pa. *November 18.*

Butterworth, K. (1979). Unwritten classroom presentation to class of graduate students at United States International University. *April 1.*

Coigney, V. (1981). Coming home - again (a play for living). Resource material from the Navy Family Support Program Division, Department of the Navy, Washington, D.C.

Cove, L.A., Fagen, S.A., & Baker, S.L. (1969). Military families in crisis. Father goes to war. Proceedings of the 46th Annual Meeting of the American Orthopsychiatric Association. *March 30-April 2.*

Cretekos, C.J. (1971). Common psychological syndromes of the army wife. Presented at the 124th annual meeting of the American Psychiatric Association, Washington, D.C. *May 3-7.*

Crumley, F.E., & Blumenthal, R.S. (1973). Children's reactions to temporary loss of the father. *American Journal of Psychiatry. 130,* 778-782.

den Dulk, D.E., & Hunter, E.J. (1981). Military enforced separations: ministering to the marital and family readjustment needs of the deployed navy men returning home. Doctoral Dissertation, San Francisco Theological Seminary, San Anselm, Ca. *June.*

Dickerson, W.J. & Arthur, R.J. (1965). Navy families in distress. *Military Medicine. 130,* 894-898.

Ebbert, J. (1980). Underway! How three commands are providing support services to navy families. Resource material from the Navy Family Support Division, Department of the Navy, Washington, D.C. *March.*

Family Program Support Division, Department of the Navy. (1981). Backgrounder: Navy Family Support Program. Resource material. Washington, D.C. *September.*

Girard, D. (1982). Clinical social workers as primary prevention agents. N.A.S.W. Clinical Symposium, Washington, D.C. *November.*

Gonzalez, V.R. (1970). *Psychiatry and the Army Brat.* Springfield, Ill.: Charles C. Thomas.

Groth A.H., Hobson, W.F., & Gary, T.S. (1982). The child molester: clinical observations. *Social Work and Child Sexual Abuse.* New York: The Haworth Press.

Kovalesky-McLaine, L. (1982). Child sexual abuse in the military family: road block or recovery? Resource material from the Navy Family Support Program Division, Department of the Navy, Washington, D.C. *May.*

Lagrone, D.M. (1978). The military family syndrome. *American Journal of Psychiatry. 135,* 1040-1043.

Lester, M. (1977). When daddy comes home. *The Chaplain. 4,* 35-41.

Lexier, L.J. (1981). The problems of father absence: a preventive program. Resource material from the Family Support Program Division, Department of the Navy, Washington, D.C. *May.*

Navy Family Support Program Division. (1981). Backgrounder: Navy Family Support Program. Resource material from the Department of the Navy, Washington, D.C. *September.*

Parry, J.S. & Parkenson, K.L. (1981). Institute on social services for military families. N.A.S.W. Professional Symposium, Philadelphia, Pa. *November.*

Pearlman, C.A., Jr. (1970). Separation reactions of married women. *American Journal of Psychiatry. 126,* 946-950.

Yeatman, G.W. (1981). Paternal separation and the military dependent child. *Military Medicine. 146,* 320-322.

A Behavioral Approach
to Time-Limited Groups

Martin Sundel
Sandra Stone Sundel

ABSTRACT. A time-limited model for behavior modification with groups is presented. The basic features and relevant techniques of the model are applied to assessment, planning, intervention and evaluation. Issues in group functioning are examined in relation to optimal performance of the group in addressing the concerns of its members. Research findings using this model in several settings are discussed. Various applications of the model are presented, including implications for future development.

Emphasis on a knowledge-based, empirical approach to social work with groups has expanded during the past decade (Lawrence and Sundel, 1972, 1975; Lawrence and Walter, 1978; Rose, 1972, 1977, 1980; Sundel and Lawrence, 1970, 1974, 1977). Social workers have become increasingly interested in the application of behavioral principles and techniques to group settings. The emphasis on accountability within the context of limited resources has fostered attempts to provide services to clients within brief time frames (Budman, 1981).

The purpose of this paper is to present a time-limited behavioral group work model and describe its application to various settings and populations. The main features of the model are reviewed, emphasizing the planning, intervention and evaluation components. Various aspects of this model have been described in the literature (Lawrence and Sundel, 1972; Lawrence and Walter, 1978; Sundel and Lawrence, 1970, 1974, 1977).

Martin Sundel, PhD, is a Roy E. Dulak Professor, Graduate School of Social Work, The University of Texas at Arlington, Arlington, Texas. Sandra Stone Sundel, MSSW is at the Jewish Social Service Agency, Fort Worth, Texas.

An earlier version of this paper was presented to the Social Work Group for the Study of Behavioral Methods at the 16th Annual Convention of the Association for the Advancement of Behavior Therapy, November 20, 1982, Los Angeles, California.

This model of group work combines the application of behavior modification principles with small group theory to pursue the specific goals of group members. In this model, the client becomes a member of the group to solve a problem of concern to the person or significant others. The objective is to change the behavior of each member outside the group where the problem occurs. Group functioning objectives, such as cohesiveness, leadership, or self-disclosure are pursued specifically to help participants achieve their goals. These group process objectives are secondary, although necessary, to the pursuit of individual goals. The behaviors that constitute appropriate participation of a group member are specified at the start of the group. Group members are expected to perform certain behaviors that contribute to optimum group functioning while they work on their own goals.

Client problems treated in this type of group have included job stress, marital discord, child management, depression, self control, anxiety, and interpersonal difficulties with friends, families, work associates, and superiors. Treatment groups typically consist of five to seven individuals. The usual course of treatment in these groups involves one individual intake session and eight weekly group sessions. Followup interviews are held one month and three or six months after termination of the group.

The group serves as the context in which the behavioral change goals of each member are pursued. The practitioner influences the activities and relationships of group members to facilitate the achievement of client objectives. The practitioner establishes group functioning goals to optimize appropriate participation of group members.

This time-limited behavioral group approach structures service delivery in order to achieve the following client objectives and group participation conditions:

1. Treatment norms are established within the group as follows: (a) Members are expected to attend every session, (b) socialization among members outside of meetings is discouraged, (c) discussion of members' problems focuses on current events and observable data, and (d) members are required to perform assignments outside the group.
2. Members prioritize their problems and establish behavioral change goals.
3. Members help each other in the assessment of their problems.

4. Members contribute suggestions for change and solutions to each other's problems.
5. Members participate actively in role playing and educational procedures designed to teach problem-solving skills.
6. Members provide social reinforcement and constructive feedback to each other.

Overview of Model

This model is based on a treatment planning cycle which has four components: assessment, planning, intervention, and evaluation. This logical, problem-solving framework requires systematically working through each phase of the cycle for each problem while managing the group process, an approach consistent with the model developed by Robert Vinter and his colleagues at the University of Michigan (Glasser, Sarri, and Vinter, 1974).

The groups have been composed of men and women ranging in age from 20-54. The groups described in this paper met for two and one-half hours once a week for eight consecutive weeks and were led by cotherapists. Other groups using this model, however, have been conducted by a single therapist.

Time-Limited Focus

The model presented here is for an eight-week group treatment program. The model was designed to be time-limited for several reasons:

1. Clients are given the expectation that their problems can be resolved in the specified period of time if they follow the prescribed procedures. If no time limits are imposed, clients could remain in the group for an indefinite period of time without making significant progress towards problem resolution. The attractiveness of group membership and participation could outweigh the incentive for clients to solve their problems quickly.
2. Clients and practitioners are encouraged to organize their group time, and to work on problem-solving activities between group sessions. Clients learn to apply principles taught in the group to their real-life problems. Managing the group process, although necessary, is secondary to the focus on problem-

solving. If problems in group functioning (for example, clique formation or scapegoating) impeded goal progress, therapists actively intervene to refocus the group. Group members become highly task-oriented in order to make the most of the time spent in group sessions.

3. Practitioners can treat more clients. By treating clients' problems within a brief interval, practitioners become available to treat more clients than is possible with long-term groups. Time-limited groups also reduce the cost of individual treatment as well as the length of suffering.

4. The behavior modification approach typically involves highly focused, goal-directed sessions that systematically work through the treatment planning cycle (Sundel and Sundel, 1982). Establishing a specific time limit for group treatment is consistent with this approach.

The time limit of eight weeks was established based on the therapists' experience of the time required to teach group participants basic problem-solving concepts for assessing and treating their problems and evaluating the outcomes. The number of sessions could be varied, however, according to the characteristics of particular groups, such as size of group, length of sessions, number of therapists, and similarity of client problems.

Assessment

Intake. Prospective group members are interviewed individually to determine the appropriateness of group treatment for their problems. The purpose of this initial interview is to identify problems that are appropriate for time-limited group treatment, and to obtain several concrete examples. During this meeting, the prospective member also agrees to follow the rules governing the group's operation.

RAC-S. In order to learn problem solving skills, group members are first taught a method for assessing problem behaviors (Lawrence and Sundel, 1972; Sundel and Sundel, 1982). This method, referred to as RAC-S, includes the following components: (1) Response; (2) Antecedents; (3) Consequences; and (4) Strength. The specification of these four elements is required of each member during the assessment phase. Assessment objectives, therefore, require each member to provide:

1. a clear definition of the problem, indicating undesired responses, their antecedents and consequences, and,
2. measures of the strength of problem behaviors, using response rate or duration data.

For example, John complained that his wife didn't understand him. The therapists and group members asked him to describe a typical incident involving him and his wife, including what each of them said and did in that situation. They continued to ask him questions until he specified his undesired response (R), its antecedents (A) and consequences (C).

One of John's problematic responses was that he continued to read the newspaper (R) when his wife asked him how his day had gone (A). As a result, she screamed at him until he put the newspaper down and yelled back (C). John was given an assignment to record the number and duration of such incidents during the next week (S).

Behavioral reenactment is a role-playing technique used to obtain RAC-S information regarding a client's behaviors in the problematic situation by observing the client role play an incident that simulates the problem. This technique is effective in a group setting because it can help the group pinpoint discrepancies between the member's report of the behavior and what is actually observed in the role play. For example, a behavioral reenactment of John's problematic situation revealed that he kept his head down and eyes focused on the newspaper when his wife asked him questions about work. There was a scowl on his face and when he finally put the paper down, he threw it on the floor.

Planning and Intervention

After RAC-S assessment data are collected, treatment goals are formulated with each member. Group members contribute to the goal statements of a member based on reported RAC-S data, as well as on observations of the individual's interactions in the group and in behavioral reenactments. Although a goal might be stated initially in broad terms, it is delineated into behaviorally specific components including desired responses (R), antecedents (A), and consequences (C).

For example, John's goal stated that when his wife asks him questions about his work (A), he would put down the newspaper, look at her and answer her questions (R). The potential positive consequences would be avoiding arguments and having pleasant conversations (C). This scenario should occur in the evenings when John comes home from work and sits down to read the newspaper. An alternative goal to be negotiated might be that when John arrives home from work (A), he asks his wife to allow him 20 minutes to read the newspaper in silence (R), after which he initiates pleasant conversation with her (C).

Behavioral change goals indicate the direction in which certain behaviors are to be modified. Behavioral techniques can be applied so that a behavior is (1) acquired or established, (2) increased in frequency, (3) maintained at a certain rate or pattern, or (4) decreased in frequency (Sundel and Sundel, 1982). One or more behavioral techniques may be included in the client's intervention plan.

The intervention plan provides a framework for systematically carrying out the behavioral change program to attain the client's goals. This plan is designed to alter behaviors and their controlling antecedents and consequences in order to move the client toward goal attainment. Without an explicit plan, application of an isolated behavioral technique could be ineffective in achieving the client's goal.

After the desired behaviors are specified in treatment goals, each member is instructed on how to perform them. Members practice these behaviors in the group, with feedback from the practitioners and other group members. Additional instructions, prompts, and cueing are given to help shape appropriate behaviors. These behavioral rehearsals allow group members to practice desired behaviors in a controlled environment until they appear competent to perform them outside the group.

A major advantage of the group is the availability of individuals who can serve as models in performing desired behaviors. Multiple models provide diverse examples of how desired behaviors can be performed and allow the group member to imitate the model that is most acceptable. Another advantage is that group members provide reinforcement to each other for appropriate behaviors. This can be more effective than if only the practitioners were providing the reinforcement. The practitioners serve as role models for group members by performing desired behaviors, as well as by demonstrating how to provide instructions, cues and positive reinforcement.

After members have demonstrated desired behaviors in the group, they are assigned to perform them in their natural environments. These tasks or behavioral assignments involve behaviors to be performed by the client outside the group setting between sessions. They are used to provide continuity between the group setting and the natural environment. They also help structure the time between group sessions so that group members can continue to work toward their treatment goals.

A significant feature of this behavioral group model is the explicit, systematic treatment planning framework that outlines the objectives and tasks to be accomplished during the group meetings. In order to pursue group maintenance and treatment goals, the practitioners prepare objectives prior to each meeting. A session-by-session plan specifies what is to be accomplished during meetings, including behaviors each member is expected to perform and interventions that could be used to achieve these objectives. This plan is revised on the basis of weekly evaluations of the group's progress. Session plans are sufficiently flexible to allow the practitioners to respond spontaneously to unexpected events.

The eight-week group treatment model was designed to implement individual treatment programs for clients. The eight sessions were carefully planned to involve the members in the following four processes:

1. *Development of group norms.* The practitioners establish rules for participation and model appropriate behavioral techniques to foster pro-treatment behaviors in the group.
2. *Education.* The practitioners teach basic principles of behavioral assessment and modification to participants and teach them how to apply these principles to their individual problems and circumstances.
3. *Problem-solving.* The practitioners lead the group in systematically assessing the problems of each member, formulating relevant goals, prescribing viable solutions, monitoring progress, and evaluating outcomes of interventions.
4. *Behavioral training and practice.* The practitioners teach group members how to perform desired behaviors using modeling, prompting, shaping, behavioral rehearsal, corrective feedback, and reinforcement. Clients practice these behaviors in the group before trying them out in the natural environment. Group members also participate in behavioral training by serv-

ing as significant others in role plays, serving as models, providing corrective feedback and suggesting alternative behaviors.

Planning for Group Meetings

In treatment groups, co-therapists have certain advantages over a
single therapist. While one therapist assumes the active role, the
other attends to the nonverbal behaviors of group members and
manages the group process. The therapists switch roles periodically
so that each one has a chance to observe and manage the group process. The leader who is observing analyzes interactions among
members and instigates changes to affect the group's functioning or
problem-solving activities. If the therapist who is the active leader
misses an important statement or nonverbal behavior, the other
therapist can pick up on it. Other benefits of co-leadership are that
group members have two professional role models in addition to
models provided by group members, a second professional's perspective on their problems, and an additional source of reinforcement. Because of the intensity of the two and one-half hour sessions
and the detailed information covered in each session, the presence
of compatible co-therapists is desirable to keep the group focused on
productive activities. In describing his model of behavioral group
therapy, Flowers (1979) indicated that two leaders were required.

Time-limited groups require ongoing monitoring by the co-therapists to ensure that sufficient time is allocated to address each member's problems. The time limitation makes it necessary for the co-
therapists to plan carefully and prioritize the activities to be covered
by the group in particular sessions. In order for the practitioners to
coordinate their efforts effectively, they plan an agenda before
group meetings and analyze the results of each meeting. The planning sessions involve discussions of each member's progress both as
a group member and as a problem-solver. Objectives for each group
meeting are established. The activities and roles of each therapist
are specified, including which therapist will begin the session, the
kinds of role plays the co-therapists will structure, and the behaviors
or techniques they will model and reinforce. In discussing each
member's progress and participation in the group, the co-therapists
also plan intervention strategies for modifying member behaviors
that impede individual or group functioning.

Co-therapists typically establish operating rules that govern their behavior in group sessions. These rules include procedures for handling differences of opinion between co-therapists during group meetings, structuring role plays and assignments, and making educational presentations.

The first two group sessions focus on problem identification and assessment of individual behaviors, establishment of problem-solving norms in the group, and presentation of basic principles of behavioral analysis. During sessions three and four, behavioral assessments are completed for all members. Intervention plans are established and implemented for individuals whose assessments were completed in previous sessions. Sessions five through seven focus on behavioral training, and assignments are given for members to implement desired behaviors in their natural environments. Session eight is devoted to evaluating member achievements in regard to goal attainment, and to scheduling follow-up meetings.

Some typical objectives for the sessions are given below:

Session 1: Objectives:
1. Each member states his or her problem in behavioral terms and gives examples specifying undesired behaviors.
2. Each member identifies an undesired behavior to observe and count during the next week.
3. Each member participates in determining problem priorities for other members.

The practitioners structure the first session to establish the clients' expectations for participation in the group. Group members are shown how to assume an active role in analyzing their problems as well as in helping other individuals to problem-solve. The task-oriented requirements for participation in the group are explained in relation to the time limits of each session as well as the overall program.

Session 2: Objectives:
1. Each member reports data from the recording assignment.
2. Each member identifies target responses, their controlling antecedents and consequences, and devises a procedure to measure response strength.
3. Each member participates in assessment activities and provides appropriate social reinforcement to other group members.

Sessions 3 and 4: Objectives:
1. Each member reports data from the assignments.

2. Each member presents examples of target responses and their strength (frequency and duration data), and controlling conditions.
3. Each member specifies a behavioral change goal and identifies examples of positive and negative reinforcement contingencies from his or her data.
4. Each member participates in prescribing intervention strategies for members who have provided sufficient assessment data.

Sessions 5-7: Objectives:
1. Each member reports data from the assignments.
2. Each member evaluates progress towards goal attainment.
3. Each member performs behavioral tasks and assignments designed to achieve his or her goals.
4. Group members participate in role plays and give each other feedback on their performances.

Session 8: Objectives:
1. Each member evaluates his or her progress towards attainment of treatment goals.
2. Each member describes a procedure for maintaining his or her treatment gains.
3. Follow-up interviews are arranged.

In order to accomplish individual goals, the practitioners take an active role in controlling group functioning so that all members have a chance to participate in problem-solving and group maintenance activities. Potential pitfalls include domination by one person, overworking one person's problem to the neglect of others, detailed discussion of irrelevant or tangential topics, inability of a member to focus on his or her problem, and non-compliance with group norms.

Evaluation

Evaluating treatment progress is based on the extent to which the client's goals are accomplished. This is determined by observation of treatment-related behaviors in the group as well as client self-evaluation reports.

In evaluating the efficacy of a behavioral change program, the practitioners consider the client's evaluation of the program's success, as well as the evaluation of significant others such as family, friends, and referral source. Measures of the client's satisfaction with the results should be consistent with his or her attainment of the treatment goals. Measures of satisfaction from clients and significant others obtained after intervention can be compared with their assessment of the target behaviors prior to implementation of the behavioral change plan, to determine their perceptions of the extent of change and the benefits of group treatment.

The practitioners discuss objective measures of progress toward goal achievement with the client and relate these measures to the client's personal satisfaction with behavioral change. Measures of client satisfaction are obtained throughout the behavioral change program so that both objective measures of goal progress and the client's perceptions of improvement can be compared. If the client's goals are achieved but the client is dissatisfied, this may indicate a failure to have established goals that are considered significant by the client. It might also mean that other problem areas need to be considered in the client's behavioral change program.

On the other hand, a client who has difficulty achieving behavioral change goals may report satisfaction with the behavioral change program. This individual may be deriving sufficient reinforcement from the relationship with the practitioner to compensate for lack of goal progress. The practitioner should help the client to realistically evaluate progress toward attainment of treatment goals and separate this evaluation from the client's satisfaction with his or her relationship with the practitioner (Sundel and Sundel, 1982).

Follow-up interviews were held with each group member individually. These sessions were designed to: (1) evaluate the extent to which treatment gains had been maintained; (2) provide additional interventions if necessary for the problem worked on during group treatment; (3) determine if additional treatment was necessary for problems not dealt with in the group or that had developed after termination of group treatment; and (4) determine if the clients had applied the techniques they learned in the group to other problems.

Research Findings

In an exploratory study using this model with three groups, 15 of the 17 (88%) group members rated their problems "much better" or "completely solved" six months after treatment. In addition, 12 of the 17 (71%) reported that they had successfully applied the behavioral concepts they learned in the group to other problems (Lawrence and Sundel, 1972; Sundel and Lawrence, 1977).

Lawrence and Walter (1978) used a controlled outcome study to further test the group model with clients in a family service agency and a community mental health clinic. These clients presented inter-personal problems with family members, acquaintances and work associates. Forty-eight subjects were randomly assigned to two conditions: the behavioral group model or a no-treatment control group. The experimental condition consisted of four groups of five or six members. Each group was led by two therapists. Subjects in the control group were placed on a waiting list until evaluation post-tests were administered nine weeks later. The behavioral group model was implemented over an eight-week period. The control group then received the same treatment.

The behavioral group model was found to be more effective than no treatment ($x^2 = 12.60$, df $= 1$, p $< .001$) according to a problem rating form filled out by each client, as well as ratings by two judges. Changes from pre-test to post-test were observed to be greater within the treatment group than within the control group on a number of other measures used (a behavioral problem-solving test, the Rathus Assertiveness Scale (1973), and two social effectiveness tests). A three-month follow-up survey of treated clients showed that 74% of the clients sustained substantial improvement.

Conclusion

Since first reported (Sundel and Lawrence, 1970), the behavioral group treatment model has been applied to a wide range of populations, including prisoners, drug addicts, mental patients, alcoholics, married couples, juvenile offenders, and non-assertive individuals. The model has been applied in out-patient mental health clinics, psychiatric hospitals, parent training seminars, and assertiveness training groups (Sundel and Sundel, 1980). Many of these groups have been conducted in practice settings, rather than under controlled experimental conditions. Unpublished and informal reports by practitioners, however, have shown the model, with minor variations, to be applicable to many populations and diverse settings.

We have described a time-limited behavioral group model and its applications to various settings and populations. The assessment-treatment planning-intervention-evaluation framework provides a problem-solving method for applying behavior modification principles with time-limited groups. Knowledge of group dimensions (for example, cohesiveness, communication patterns) and related group management skills (for example, establishing and enforcing group norms) are essential in directing group activities toward achievement of individual goals. Future research in the use of this model could focus on evaluative comparisons with other short-term group models, determining the optimum composition and duration of groups for differing client populations and problems, and assessing the impact of time-limited groups on the productivity and operation of social agencies.

REFERENCES

Budman, S.H. (Ed.). (1981). *Forms of brief therapy.* New York: Guilford Press.
Flowers, J.V. (1979). Behavioral analysis of group therapy and a model for behavioral group therapy. In D. Upper & S. Ross, (Eds.), *Behavioral group therapy.* Champaign, Ill.: Research Press.
Glasser, P., Sarri, R., & Vinter, R. (Eds.). (1974). *Individual change through small groups.* New York: The Free Press.
Lawrence, H., & Sundel, M. (1972). Behavior modification in adult groups. *Social Work, 17*(2), 34-43.
Lawrence, H., & Sundel, M. (1975). Self-modification in groups: A student training method for social groupwork. *Journal of Education for Social Work, 11*(2), 76-83.
Lawrence, H., & Walter, C. (1978). Testing a behavioral approach with groups. *Social Work, 23*(2), 127-133.
Rathus, S.A. (1973). A 30-item schedule for assessing assertive behavior. *Behavior Therapy, 4,* 398-406.
Rose, S. (1972). *Treating children in groups.* San Francisco: Jossey-Bass.
Rose, S. (1977). *Group therapy: A behavioral approach.* Englewood Cliffs, N.J.: Prentice-Hall, Inc.
Rose, S. *A casebook in group therapy.* Englewood Cliffs, N.J.: Prentice-Hall, Inc.
Sundel, M., & Lawrence, H. (1970). Time-limited behavioral group treatment with adults. *Michigan Mental Health Research Bulletin, 4,* 37-40.
Sundel, M., & Lawrence, H. (1974). Behavioral group treatment with adults in a family service agency. In P. Glasser, R. Sarri, & R. Vinter (Eds.), *Individual change through small groups.* New York: The Free Press.
Sundel, M., & Lawrence, H. (1977). A systematic approach to treatment planning in time-limited behavioral groups. *Journal of Behaviour Therapy and Experimental Psychiatry, 8,* 395-399.
Sundel, M., & Sundel, S. (1982). *Behavior modification in the human services: A systematic introduction to concepts and applications.* Second Edition. Englewood Cliffs, N.J.: Prentice-Hall, Inc.
Sundel, S.S., & Sundel M. (1980). *Be Assertive: A Practical Guide for Human Service Workers.* Beverly Hills, CA: Sage.

PRACTICE NOTES

The notes that follow provide brief pragmatic illustrations of practice which consciously *uses* limited time as an independent variable that can affect the outcome of group experience. Alternatively, these workers recognize time-limited groups as the *matrix* for their helping services. The selections are representative of differing populations in diverse settings with a wide range of purposes. A variety of practice orientations and interventions are also presented.

Almost without exception, these notes were excerpted and edited from full presentations that are rich in bibliographic support for the worker's rationale. Regrettably, space does not permit publication here of the complete works. Even this limitation can be viewed as an asset, however. It led the editors to focus these "notes" on the inductive approach, which starts with the empirical world, rather than the more common deductive approach which starts with hypotheses and conceptual frameworks (as we did in the first section of this volume).

Reader's, therefore, are urged to examine these practice notes carefully and to compare the practices described here with their own experiences.

AEROBIC THERAPY:
A FEMINIST/WHOLISTIC APPROACH
IN TIME-LIMITED GROUP PRACTICE

An innovative approach in time-limited group practice is available through aerobic therapy. Aerobic exercise has been defined as vigorous physical exertion using the large muscle groups within arms and legs, which maintain the heart rate at 70% to 85% of its maximum level for at least twenty minutes. In order to experience the positive outcomes associated with aerobic exercise, persons must engage within that type of activity at least three times per week. Both theoretical perspectives and empirical findings suggest that a regular regimen of aerobic exercise can have significant implications in reducing depression, anxiety, stress and other negative mental health indicators. The practice model described here involves the utilization of aerobic exercise and group psychotherapy in mediating nonpsychotic, negative mental health indicators.

The aerobic therapy group meets for two hours, once a week, for a ten week period. The first hour is devoted to exercise, commencing with a 15 minute warm-up. Anerobic exercises which include stretching and strengthening approaches are utilized in order to prepare participants for the more strenuous, subsequent component. During stretching, instrumental music is played to enhance enjoyment of the activity and group leaders facilitate light conversation in order to add humor as well as encouragement for exercising. At the end of the warm-up, music is switched to "up-beat" mode so that participants can accelerate their heart beat rate to 70%-80% of the maximum for their age group. To determine one's aerobic rate, the following formula is provided:

Formula	*Example*
a) 220	220
$\underline{- \text{ age of participant}}$	$\underline{- \;\; 40}$ (age)
remainder	180
b) $\underline{\times \; .80}$	$\underline{\times \; .80}$
maximum heart rate	144.00 heart beats per minute
for 60 seconds	$144 \div 10 = 14.4$
$\div 10 =$	pulse beats per 6 seconds

c) maximum heart rate

For the aerobic component, participants set off in groups of at least two, to either walk, walk/jog or jog for 30 minutes. It is helpful to run this type of group with 2 co-therapists, as each can take responsibility for overseeing different aerobic participation levels. This part of the group provides an excellent opportunity for bonding and personal sharing since participants chat with each other as they exercise.

Subsequent to being aerobic, there is a ten minute "cool down" where members do stretching exercises. The purpose of this activity is to lengthen muscles which have become oxygenated through exercise. It also provides a way for members to control their breathing and relax.

Participants are encouraged to engage in aerobic activity, including warm-ups and cool-downs, at least twice a week outside of the group. This is to encourage development of the maximum aerobic effect.

For the last hour, there is group dialogue on topics germane to depression and stress, such as: helplessness, loss, guilt, role expectations, relationships, cognitive distortions, etc. Each member of the group is asked to speak on the chosen topic, briefly, in round-robin fashion in order to ensure all participants articulate on the theme. Subsequently, in-depth discussion is encouraged. As is true with any group, care must be given that certain participants do not monopolize the conversation. The utility of this approach, especially for women, is that participants share many common experiences in what generates depression/stress for them, regardless of being homemakers or paid workers. That is, they learn that their experience is not unique, that they are not alone and that their feelings are not "wrong." Additionally, participants have many coping strategies to share with each other; particularly in terms of how they have dealt with child rearing and relationship issues.

The co-therapists act in facilitative roles as well as to share information in a re-educative therapeutic approach. For example, the concept of "cognitive distortions" would be explained; participants would then be asked to talk about the pertinence of those phenomena for themselves.

It needs to be emphasized that this approach works best with a more homogeneous population. Experience has shown that persons who perceive themselves as dissimilar from other group members, drop-out. Also, although there are cross-generational similarities shared by women, such as expectations related to nurturing and care-taking, those closer in age have had more comparable opportunities which enhances group dialogue.

It should be emphasized that the reason this particular approach has focused on women is that traditional sex role socialization tends to dissuade females from evolving their physical selves. The healthy male is one of sound mind and body, so speaks stereotypes; yet, women are not encouraged to be assertive in any mode. Although this model suggests particular import for women, it could be utilized with a variety of population groups. For example, it would be an excellent approach to use with senior citizens, abusive spouses/parents, stressed-out professionals/business executives, acting-out children, etc.

In order to ascertain if this approach is effective in reducing depression and stress, evaluative criteria have been included. The Beck Depression Inventory as well as the Quick Stress Index (both Likert-format assessments) have been given in order to generate pregroup/postgroup comparison data. The former measure ascertains depressive attitudes as well as behavioral indicators; whereas, the latter instrument assesses stress related to nutrition, emotions, use of substances, physical condition, environmental conditions, time management, paid employment and life changes.*

Additionally, participants are encouraged to monitor themselves daily on their level of depression, stress and participation in exercise. This is done through a graphed single subject design format as noted in Figure 1. Besides providing an additional means by which to determine the effectiveness of this approach for individual clients, daily monitoring can increase awareness of precipitators to depression/stress. Also, charting on a regular basis can be empowering by providing clients with feedback on their progress in feeling better.

Implications for Time-Limited Treatment

There are a variety of reasons why the time-limited format of this approach is functional. First of all, a cognitively-oriented treatment model has been found to be effective in short-term therapy when dealing with depression. By highlighting a client's cognitive distortions and pinpointing the feelings as well as behaviors associated with those dysfunctional thoughts, clients can modify cognitions and experience positive change/within a relatively short period of time.

Secondly, this ten week group emphasizes acquiring self-help skills which can be employed by the individual subsequently, and

---

*The Beck Depression Inventory is a 21 item, 4 category Likert assessment which has been empirically substantiated as a reliable and valid index for measuring depression. For information on its construction, scoring and utilization, see David Burns, *Feeling Good,* New York, Signet, 1981, pp. 19-27. The Quick Stress Index is an, as yet, unstandardized assessment, organized in Likert format, which assesses stress as a multidimensional variable. For copies of this assessment, please contact: Janet Lapp, PhD, Associate Professor, Department of Psychology, California State University, Fresno, Fresno, CA 93740.

Figure 1

Single Subject Design Graphs for Daily
Monitoring of Depression, Stress and
Exercise

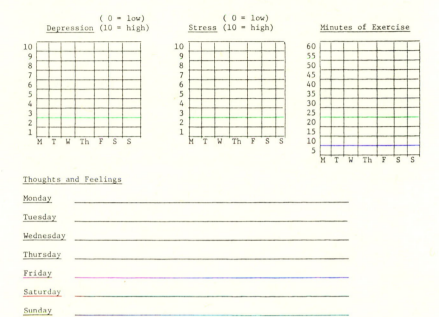

generalized to coping with distress in the future. There is a certain sense of immediacy in following through with a personal aerobic exercise plan while there is an opportunity for feedback from group facilitators.

Thirdly, operating from a time-limited group format allows for sharing a greater amount of information than might be accomplished within individual psychotherapy sessions. In other words, this model has a more educative format than is the norm in more traditional approaches. Also, clients learn a significant amount from each other in terms of coping strategies which would not be available through individual treatment.

Forthly, in that participants understand that the group is short-term, there can be a greater investment in trying to maximally gain from the experience. That is, members may be more willing to embark upon a personal exercise regimen outside of the group or to share their feelings. In terms of the latter, an impetus is provided to deal with personal distress that might generally be placed on the "back burner." In essence, a short-term group provides a subtle pressure to deal with issues clients might usually try to avoid.

Fifthly, in terms of resource expenditures, clients may be more able to commit both time and money when a therapeutic modality is seen as time-limited. Counseling can be an expensive venture, so that a therapy which is known to be short-term may be perceived as potentially more cost-effective, by clients. Additionally, because of the multiple life roles and responsibilities which may accrue to participants, committing time for an experience that is short-term might seem more feasible. This could be particularly salient for employed persons.

Finally, by participating in a time-limited experience perceived as beneficial by a client, s/he may be more willing to become involved in future short-term "self-improvement" ventures. As a testimony to this potential, one group member decided, by virtue of her aerobic group participation, that she would enroll in an adult education assertiveness training class. It became apparent to her that much could be gained, in terms of personal rewards, by investing in a time-limited experience. (*Edited.*)

Submitted by:
Nan Van Den Bergh
Department of Social Work Education
California State University

ADMINISTRATIVE ASSISTANTS
IN THE PUBLIC SCHOOL:
THE UNDERUTILIZED RESOURCE

In various schools throughout the country, especially during the past fifteen years, a new staff position has been created for security purposes. The person who fills this position is most often an untrained non-professional who has a genuine interest in youth and who becomes known by a variety of official, unofficial and, at times, pejorative titles. Depending upon who is doing the talking, the job titles include: administrative assistant, supervisory aide, hall or lunchroom monitor, cop and "narc" (narcotics squad). Whatever the title might be, these people are clearly hired to perform a "police-like" function.

Despite their apparent one-dimensional purpose, the assistants are implicitly called upon to provide a more complex, valuable and difficult service. The juggling of roles which they must assume is, in itself, a formidable challenge. To be a friend and authority to the students, a support to teachers and an arm of the administration requires extraordinary flexibility and solid grounding. The most experienced of so-called "human relations" workers should be baffled by the contradictions inherent in the job. Their undifferentiated role precipitates much confusion and frustration and ultimately leads to a lessening of job satisfaction and to a diminution of performance, hence output is curtailed.

A partnership between a Child Guidance Center and a local school system resulted in a project in which Administrative Assistants employed by the school district were trained by Guidance Center staff. The purpose of the training, based upon a group work model was to enhance job satisfaction and to improve the overall quality of service to the school district.

The conceptual framework for the project centered on: (1) "the group-in situation as the unit of attention" and (2) short term group work. The focus was not solely on group development, but also on building environmental competence and upon creating a functional balance between autonomy and reciprocity. As the "assistant group" is described the unequal distribution of power in the school will become evident, thus the need for developing both individual competence and team work. A time limited orientation necessitated an active, conscious, ego-oriented process to define the problem and to set and achieve specific goals.

The group of "assistants" was comprised of ten members, one black male, four black females and five white females. Their ages ranged from the late twenties to early sixties and all were high school graduates. The length of time that they had been employed by the school ranged from less than one to fifteen years. The group was scheduled to meet for six sessions, one and a half hours each meeting.

The beginning phase was evidenced by a high level of suspicion and fear regarding confidentiality. The group workers (the authors) discovered that the assistants had been offered the group as a "try it, you'll like it" experience. They may have been made "an offer that they could not refuse." The ethic of self-determination seemed to be resting on uneasy ground at that point. As the group articulated their understanding of the group, meetings were transformed into something special and unique. As they came to trust the workers, they were empowered and began the task of defining themselves. The metaphors which were used and unanimously agreed upon to describe themselves revealed their sense of confusion, feelings of powerlessness and low self and collective esteem. They saw themselves as the ''bottom of the heap'' with a desire to be more than ''statues with (flailing) claws.'' These metaphors were operationalized. From this, the problem definition and goals emerged.

The group purpose arrived at was to identify, explore and problem solve around those critical issues which the assistants themselves saw as interfering with their abilities to perform the task at hand. In format, the group was to provide the context for mutual exploration and support. Critical issues were identified in three areas: (1) addressing concerns related to administrative direction, (2) improvement of the ability to intervene in situations involving students and (3) exploration of working relationships with other school staff.

As the group moved to middle phase several themes arose: (1) manifest issues regarding allegiances to students versus administrators; (2) a need for specific skill development (i.e., crisis intervention); (3) a desire to be informed of students who have special needs, (i.e., asthma, hyperactivity, epilepsy, etc.); and (4) a wish for a better feedback process with administration. The assistants struggled with numerous transferences to them: friend, cop, ''narc,'' clergyman, brother, mom, pop, therapist. This added to their confusion around the formulation of their role and the anticipation of their responses to different situations and crises. For many of the members, their identifications both inside and outside of the school system were not of an authoritarian nature. When faced with a situation of having to ''confront'' a teacher who had not complied with the rules, an internal crisis was precipitated. The crisis was further exacerbated by the unspoken expectation that the assistants should report to a group (administration) about some of that group's own members (faculty). This double-bind dynamic arose frequently. There was great relief when the group members discovered that, in some way, all of them shared such experiences. This enabled them to better understand and cope with some of the more difficult feelings that were related to their job.

In the ending phase, early suspicion gave way to trust which led to revelation, differentiation and problem solving. This stage involved an exploration of the steps which would be necessary to better integrate the assistants group into the whole of the school system. This theme appropriately led into the process of ending and re-entry. The group decided to call for a seventh and final meeting which was to include selected assistant representatives, the principal who was the broker responsible for arranging the project, the assistants' supervisor and the two workers.

There was great anticipation leading up to the intergroup meeting. The original anxieties regarding trust and confidentiality re-emerged. This regression was related to both the ending and to realistic concerns regarding the face-to-face, heart-to-heart that was being planned with their "bosses." The aim of the meeting was to evaluate the project and to share specific concerns and requests with the administration. Their anxiety was reduced as an agenda was set, thus partializing their thoughts and feelings. Three delegates were chosen and four issues were outlined. These issues were: (1) to improve staff uniformity in the enforcement of the student disciplinary code; (2) to improve the coverage at special problem locations in the school; (3) to arrange for the assistants, when appropriate, to be apprised of students with special needs (i.e., medical); (4) to continue some form of group training.

The most salient feature of the seventh meeting was the revelation that the two administrators, middle management in the school hierarchy, were also victims of the lack of uniformity around rules. They revealed their own frustration with the powers above them and for a moment the so called "bottom of the heap" seemed a bit more crowded.

In evaluating the group experience the assistants reported improved morale, increased understanding of the "chain of command" and decision making processes, less ambiguity and greater group cohesion. In addition, judging from the seventh meeting, the inter-group communication had improved. (*Edited.*)

Submitted by:
Andrew Malekoff, ACSW
Suburban Family Life Center Coordinator
North Shore Child Guidance Center
Manhasset, NY

Martin Golloub, CSW
Private Practice
Glen Cove, NY

BRIDGING THE ISOLATION GAP:
MAKING A TELEPHONE CONNECTION

Over the years, colleges have seen an increase of disabled students. The setting for this project was the Brooklyn Center of Long
Island University. The University's Special Educational Services
Program provides a range of supportive services to disabled
students, including academic, vocational and social work counseling. For LIU, this disabled population also includes people who are
homebound. These students attend classes by way of telephone lines
which directly connect their residences with the classroom. For a
number of years an intercom system was used in which an intercom
box had to be transported to each of the student's classes and placed
on the professor's desk. This box connected the classroom to
another intercom box in the student's home. However, students
could not always hear clearly. Also, in order to speak, they had to
push a button which produced a loud click, and this often inhibited
their participation.

Utilizing more advanced technology, Special Educational Services Program switched to a conference phone system in 1980.
Rather than having an intercom box sit on the professor's table, tele-
phones were installed in locked cabinets within the classroom. The
professor simply dials the student's number at the beginning of the
class and plugs in a microphone so the homebound student can hear
and be heard by the other students. The reception is better, the system is more sophisticated and more personalized.

Starting in 1977, a social work group was formed as a *network for
homebound students.* The idea was to provide students with a forum
to share concerns, discuss their unique needs as homebound students, and provide a mutual support system. In managing this group
the then existing intercom boxes were used, and the worker sat at a
table with the boxes in a semicircle, allowing each student to com-
municate both with the worker and with the other students. Thus, a
group was formed without actual face-to-face contact among its
members.

With the advent of the conference phone system, the format of the
group had to be changed. Whereas with the intercom system an un-
limited number of students could be connected without incurring a
large expense, under the telephone system it was now extremely
costly to hook up more than two students at one time. Since only two
students could be on the phone at once, the idea of *dyad pairing* was

introduced. Expanding this concept, a *triad* was considered as yet another possibility, taking advantage of the fact that there is a population of homebound students able to attend some classes on campus. Having those on-campus students sit with the worker, communicating with the two on the telephone, a triad could be formed.

An initial letter of recruitment was sent to each of the School-to-Home-Network students explaining the rationale and format of the new group. It was made clear that this was not to be an ongoing group but rather individual one-session groups, and that the composition of the group and the topics could change each week. The letter was followed up by individual interviews. Recruitment interviews served two functions—the matchings were in part based on the worker's impressions, and the worker was aided to bridge the gap left by the absence of visual cues. The individual contacts were crucial to the pairing, which was based on the students' choice of topics of interest.

Each meeting involved the phases of group development in a condensed form. The purpose of both the individual group and the total project were stated at the start of each meeting. A contract for discussion and material to be covered was developed, members were engaged to participate, and at the end of the meeting they terminated through summing up and feedback.

In some ways, greater demands are placed on the worker in the single-session group because of its finality. Before the session takes place there is preparatory empathy and the worker must anticipate directions the session might take. S/he must tune-in sharply, quickly join the members together, and while remaining a facilitator, direct the flow of the discussion. Single-session groups require specialized skills: tuning-in, contracting, getting in to the work, and termination, all in one or two hours. In addition, the absence of visual contact and the lack of body and non-verbal cues heightened the need for the worker to be more acutely attuned to the verbal messages. Inasmuch as the students did not physically meet together, it was imperative that the worker create a confidential environment. At the start of each session the meeting room was described and it was made clear to all participants that only they were present, and that all material discussed would be confidential.

Regardless of the topics discussed, mutual aid and a social and helping network were fostered at all meetings. Suggestions for success as a homebound student were always offered within the context of the discussion. Students were supportive of one another, able to

share feelings, and ventilate frustrations. The group served to intro-
duce students to each other and help establish networks of people
and relationships which in turn functioned as bridges between the
person and the environment. The personal networks included persons who are connected through intermediaries to the central figure
or an "anchor" person. Students were encouraged by the worker to
exchange phone numbers and to contact one another after the group
meeting.

Each student participated once or twice, but those who took part
in two groups were never paired with the same person or persons
more than once. There was, however, a high level of participation
and involvement. The smallness of the group made it conducive for
each to participate fully. In addition, each student knew beforehand
the topic of focus for the meeting which was based on his/her own
interests which were expressed during the recruitment process.
Having been alerted by the worker regarding the commonality on
which the meeting was to be based, the students had time to organize
their thoughts and do some preparatory work. Finally, the premise
of this experiment, as conveyed to the students, was for it not to be a
static, ongoing group, and the result was that they made the most of
the single-session opportunity by participating fully.

The worker served different functions in different group meetings. Working with any type of group implies the need for flexibility
and the ability to take on a variety of roles as the situation dictates.
Within the framework of the single-session group there is even a
greater demand for the worker to assume flexible roles because
he/she never deals with the same configuration of members more
than once. The unknown factor of how members will interact requires more openness to role change. The even more specific situation of single-session groups of homebound persons conducted over
the telephone calls upon the worker to act in additional and more
flexible capacities.

The *roles* that a worker assumes during the course of the meeting
are *directly related to a moment to moment assessment* of group and
individual needs, members' responses, and feedback. The worker
takes on special roles or variations of translator, moderator, en-
abler, facilitator, mediator, change agent, resource person, and ad-
vocate. For example, one student's disability manifested halting and
unintelligible speech, making it difficult for others to know when he
has finished speaking. Another student breathed through a res-
pirator, which made his speech difficult to understand and also pre-

sented the same problem of not knowing when he was finished speaking. The worker translated for the two students with speech difficulties and often had to repeat what could not be understood. The moderator role was used frequently to "traffic" the timing of students' speech so that the slow speakers would not be interrupted.

Although this experiment was geared to a specific population, there is great potential to establish channels of communication for other individuals with common interests and concerns, who, for various reasons, cannot get together in the same physical place. These include: the elderly; persons with the same disability, chronic illness or degenerative illness; mothers at home with young children; and people in rural settings with common problems or similar interests. (*Edited.*)

Submitted by:
Ruth Pollock Shilman, MSW
Field Placement Supervisor
Long Island University
Brooklyn, NY

Beth Horowitz Giladi, MA
Special Education Consultant
Jewish Education Association
of Metro-West
New Jersey

AN ECLECTIC APPROACH TO GROUP WORK WITH THE ALCOHOLIC'S "FAMILY" SYSTEM DURING SHORT-TERM INPATIENT TREATMENT

An eclectic combination of behavioral, interactional, and structural approaches applied in both a "Family" Relations Group and a Multiple Family Group can help reach alcoholics on a short-term treatment unit.

The "family" system of the alcoholic is deemed to include significant people who are married to, live with, related to, or friends of the person with an alcohol problem. Since the alcoholic is emotionally isolated from others and tends to have only superficial and manipulative relationships with "significant" others, the integration of the present "family" system into the group work process is a crucial link during the inpatient treatment stay. This is designed to foster better mutual understanding between patients and their "family" system in order to assure the patients' continued well-being after discharge.

In terms of short-term crisis intervention work, the group worker seems to have the most impact *after* the detoxification process has been completed. Being no longer "wet," or drinking, the patient is then more accessible to begin communication with his/her "family" system, while the inpatient stay provides a key source of initial stability. The task of the worker is two fold: first to establish a Relations Group for "family" members only, *without* the patient; then to use this group as a sub-group in a total Multiple Family Group where the systems can be observed, evaluated, and worked with to offer relief from the immediate crisis.

The Relations Group, composed of the patient's "family," meets one and one half hours weekly *without* the patient, providing the opportunity for (1) asking questions, (2) expressing specific feelings and concerns, (3) examining interactional patterns and the relationships between these patterns and the drinking behavior, (4) identifying present problem areas, and (5) receiving a basic education about alcoholism.

With behavioral focus on the adaptive consequences of drinking, and nonjudgemental interactional focus on sharing and listening, the worker can help the "family" members to structurally reframe their perception of the organization of the system.

The Multiple Family Group, composed of patients and their "family" systems, also meet weekly for one and one half hours to stimulate better mutual understanding in order to assure the patients' continued well-being after discharge. The goals are: (1) to help people talk to each other in a way that will decrease the stress and tension that alcoholism causes in the family system, (2) to identify present problem areas, (3) to examine the family system's need to change, and (4) to encourage families to continue in outpatient treatment. Since participation in the Relations Group usually has decreased anxiety, "family" members are willing to talk in the Multiple Family Group about behavior and stress that has been caused by the drinking behaviors. This is extremely important for the patients to hear because frequently they will not have remembered these past intoxicated behaviors and events. The interactional group process then encourages identification of present problem areas and the systems' needs for structural change. The group worker helps the "families" with their beginning structural changes and then prepares the "families" for out-patient groups to continue this work. *(Edited.)*

Submitted by:
David J. Matulis, ACSW
V.A. Medical Center
West Haven, Connecticut

EFFECTS OF TIME LIMITATION
IN A LOW SELF-CONCEPT CHILDREN'S GROUP

The development of brief treatment groups for children can benefit from ideas borne from experience. A low self concept children's group is discussed herein in terms of how the constraint of time limitation affects the group.

The group was composed of five third-graders, three girls and two boys. The children were referred by their teacher who felt that these children were evidencing some degree of chronic low self-concept usually demonstrated by varying degrees of isolation from peers, low classroom participation, acting out, etc. The group met weekly for nine 45-minute sessions.

The purposes of the group were to improve self-concept and to promote meaningful peer relationships. These purposes were accomplished by using structured activities such as role playing, behavioral contracting, films, puppets, and discussions. The "STORE" token economy system concept was utilized to positively reinforce individual and group goal attainment and compliance with group norms.

A behavioral tracking chart, posted at the end of each of the nine sessions showing each member's name was used to record achievement in three areas: individual goal achievement, compliance with group behavioral norms, and attendance. Stars were placed beside each member's name to show accomplishment in each area at the end of every session. Every third session tokens (representing the star) were distributed and could be used as currency at the STORE to purchase small toys, trinkets, food, etc.

Self-monitoring was used to determine the member's individual goal accomplishment while a buddy system was used to monitor compliance with group behavioral norms. At the end of each session each child reported on the progress of her/his buddy and presented (or did not present) the appropriate rewards.

Pre-Group Planning and Member Selection

The leader was responsible for the group's format—including determining the number of sessions, meeting place, time, making the appropriate school contacts, meeting with parents and gaining parental permission, etc. All concerned authority figures were involved in the planning. This often included talking with the teacher, the principal, the guidance counselor, and others in order that they might understand the group's purpose and lend their support. During the pre-group phase the leader also planned the activities to be utilized in future sessions. These included such things as films, puppets, role playing activities, values clarification exercises. The leader also prepared charts for recording compliance to group behavioral norms and individual goal attainment.

A first step in the member selection process was the pre-group interview with the child, used to determine the appropriateness of the group for this individual. Other uses were to provide an explanation of the group purpose, to determine motivation of the prospective member, and to discuss individual goals. For example, in this group, a group goal was to improve socialization skills with peers, while an individual goal within the group was to learn to get along better with a sibling.

As is true in most brief treatment groups, the importance of selecting members with high motivation levels was critical. Drop-outs will be more critical to group development and outcome than in a long-term group. Because there is not enough time to replace drop-outs the group can deteriorate rapidly if members are not carefully selected.

Role of the Leader

Due to the time constraints the leader in this group had to be more active and directive especially in the beginning.

Early leader activity was necessary to:

1. Encourage setting of behavior norms. The members were asked which things they thought they should and should not do for the group to run properly and for them to benefit. The norms decided upon were: (a) no fighting, (b) only one person could talk at a time, (c) sharing of materials, (d) honestly sharing feelings, and (e) attendance (this was suggested by the leader as essential with the promise of a "perfect attendance" certificate).

2. Encourage an early understanding of the group purpose through discussion during the first session and through re-focusing on it each time the members strayed. As the group developed the members assumed this function ("checking" each other).

3. Contribute to the development of rapid group cohesion that is so essential to short-term groups. The active leader may facilitate group passage through formation and functioning by utilizing knowledge of the members gained through interviews with the children and teacher. An initial step is to help them to connect with each other by mentioning the areas in which all share concerns. Early discussions centered around similarities of problems the members were experiencing. Since several children had experienced problems related to divorce, this was an early theme. The Dr. Seuss film "The Sneetches" reinforced members' similarities in concern over being victims of exclusion and pre-judgement of others based on appearance or first impressions. Discussion emphasis was on how much we are alike underneath, how we have similar experiences and emotions which can be shared in the group, and how a non-judgemental attitude is important in the group. To exemplify this, cards with various emotions on them were passed around to each member. Each was asked to act-out the listed emotion (and later tell of a time when each had experienced the emotion). Members were asked to guess which emotion each other member was portraying.

4. Promptly recognize and deal with threats to cohesion and development such as in the following examples:

THREATS	*SOLUTIONS*
Monopolizing Member	Ignore interruptions, emphasize norm of speaking one at a time, buddy pointing out behavior's effect on the group.

THREATS	*SOLUTIONS*
Absence	Charting presence of each member, award for perfect attendance.
Sub-grouping	Discouraged by seating arrangements and pairing for activities.
Non-participation	Having group members express to the silent member their desire for her/him to participate, discuss effect of non-participation on group functioning.
Norm-breaking	When it occurs, the leader encourages discussion of its effect; e.g., talking out of turn, group loses opportunity to share feelings of others and learn about other members. Later this function is turned over to the group. Buddies monitor behavior.

Member roles included obeying norms, open participation and disclosure, functioning in the buddy role, and working on individual goals. It was also a critical role of members to transfer responsibility for the functioning of the group from the leader to themselves as quickly as possible. Because it was a short-term group this was emphasized from the very beginning.

Time-Limited Focus

The focus was more limited and goal-oriented than in long term groups. The orientation was both "here and now" and "there and then." In and out of group and past and present behaviors were discussed, but the emphasis was always on goal attainment and accomplishment of group purpose. This limited focus contributed to cohesion. Members eagerly sought out similarities in backgrounds, shared experiences, compared personalities, discussed current problems, talked about target behavior and compared goals for themselves. It appeared as though holding fewer meetings had a stabilizing effect on the group. Their awareness of time encouraged members to work quickly toward their goals.

Overall, there needs to be a high degree of structure in time-limited groups, especially children's groups. This need for structure encompasses all major components of group development, including the role of leader, role of members, focus, selection and planning. These all need to be more structured than in long-term group treatment to facilitate more rapid movement through the stages of group development and ultimately to contribute to the efficacy of treatment. *(Edited.)*

Submitted by:
Barry M. Daste, ACSW
Patricia O. Cox, MSW
Louisiana State University
School of Social Work
Baton Rouge

THE SINGLE SESSION GROUP: AN INNOVATIVE APPROACH TO THE WAITING ROOM

The development of alternative social work services for people receiving ongoing treatment in hospital out-patient departments has generated great interest recently. Small groups have been set up in hospital waiting rooms in order to counteract the alienating influence of a large system. An innovative program has recently been developed in a large tertiary care hospital where a series of single session groups were utilized to deal with the problems of isolation and passivity exhibited by patients in the waiting room. This program is particularly interesting because it capitalized on a time-limited service to a particular patient group in their own therapeutic milieu. Only a few practice examples of single session groups have been discussed in the literature.

This program was aimed at the population of insulin-dependent patients between the ages of 18 and 45, who attended the Metabolic Day Center on a regular basis. These patients were seen monthly by their doctors for urine and blood tests to ensure that their chronic illness was monitored and regulated. They arrived at the clinic in the morning and spent from 7:30 a.m. to 3:30 p.m. in the waiting room, leaving only for meals and tests. It was noticed by the clinic staff that patients did not generally speak to each other during their long stay in the waiting room. The staff also felt that they were too busy in the clinic to involve themselves more informally with the patients.

A clinical social worker, with an extensive understanding of diabetes and its social and psychological implications initiated the program and provided the direct group work service. The contract was for 8 weekly single group sessions to be held from 9:00-10:00 a.m. in a small room adjoining the waiting room. The head nurse notified the social worker before each meeting which patients (i.e., insulin dependent, 18-45 years of age, English speaking) qualified for the group. The social worker approached these patients, explained the purpose of the group and invited them to participate. Without exception, all chose to attend. The average attendance at each group session was 5, with a range from 4 to 8 members and included both males and females. During the 8 sessions, only one person attended more than one meeting. That was a woman who attended two additional sessions on her non-clinic days as part of a plan to start a self-help group for diabetics in her own suburban community.

The purpose of this group was to encourage the development of a mutual aid system and support network in the natural setting of the waiting room. Members of the group initiated discussion on topics of interest to them related to their illness. Such topics included the specifics of their illness and disclosure of it, medical complications, pregnancy, suggestions related to their diet, family support systems or lack of them, new treatments, etc. The patients used these meetings, with the worker's help, to rehearse how they could discuss their problems more effectively with their doctors. They were also interested in providing feedback about their experiences at the clinic. It is obvious that the single session group worker had to be skilled in establishing and maintaining structure, in holding the group to its purpose, and in responding only to needs of the members within a limited context. Her job was to develop a positive support system in the group even if it is just for one hour. The phases of group development often occur in a spiral-like sequence. The normal ongoing group has the opportunity to go back to earlier phases to reinforce the gains made in that stage. In this single session group, there was a very clear demarcation between each phase.

The worker, because of the time limitation, was very active in moving the group from the beginning phase through the middle phase and on to a very definite ending phase. The beginning phase was marked by a clear statement of group purpose and an invitation to every member to briefly tell his "story." The middle phase began with the worker identifying certain common concerns of diabetics in general. She then elicited responses from the group members as to whether these concerns are relevant to them as well. This initial direct intervention by the worker opens the door for members to problem swap, to expose their own feelings about their illness, to reach out to the others and to offer suggestions and advice. In this phase, the worker, after the initial thrust, occupies a less central position. However, because the group only meets once, the worker must be very sensitive to the risks the members take and must be ready to either protect a vulnerable patient or to control one who may try to take over the group. Due to the time limitation, she cannot rely on the group to do this by themselves since that ability generally develops slowly over time.

Since these members will be unlikely to attend another meeting, the worker cannot leave any issues unsettled but must make every session a complete experience. Ten minutes before the end, the worker summarizes the discussion and reiterates some positive ideas which the members can obtain from this session.

The option of reacting to "doorknob issues" by suggesting that the group could discuss it next session is not available. The worker's role is critical in helping this group move appropriately from one phase to another while at the same time creating a positive and supportive atmosphere. This is essential if members are to be encouraged to risk. The limits of time definitely have the effect of increasing the intensity of the experience. It was evident in these sessions that the members counted on the worker to provide direct help in dealing with their painful feelings. The sensitivity and skill of the worker enabled this to happen and was most significant in the overall success of the program.

The results of this single session group experience for diabetics as measured by feedback from the clinic staff and the participants were excellent. Each group differed somewhat in topics discussed but all agreed that the experience had been a helpful one. The group always ended with some members spontaneously exchanging phone numbers. The worker also encouraged them to continue talking informally to each other in the waiting room. It was interesting that no demands were made on the social worker by either the staff or the patients for additional social work services. The purpose of the group was obviously clear and accepted by all. The response of this nursing staff and the doctors was very positive due to their continued involvement by the social worker throughout the development of the program.

This type of group could prove to be useful in many situations where people share a common problem and are waiting for service. This time limited program does not require a long term commitment from either the worker or the patients and as such is a viable option in this era of cutbacks and limited resources. *(Edited.)*

Submitted by:
Tryna Rotholz
School of Social Work
McGill University
Montreal, Quebec

CHARACTERISTICS AND CONSEQUENCES OF A TIME-LIMITED WRITING GROUP IN AN ACADEMIC SETTING

Throughout the history of the social work profession, pressures produced by time limits have figured in the strategies for interventive efforts with clients. Short term groups for therapeutic purpose and for the achievement of other life tasks have been utilized by social workers from all methods. However, social workers appear to have made limited use of time-bounded groups for the attainment of their own professional objectives.

These practice notes report on a short-term task and support group of women faculty at a major metropolitan school of social work. It was organized in response to demands for academic productivity placed on faculty in times of shrinking budgets and withdrawal from affirmative action goals that had briefly expanded the opportunity structure for women and minority faculty.

The goal of the group was to increase individual scholarly work, a format for productivity which contrasts with traditional collaborative efforts. Composition, setting and expectations were designed to further the productivity goal. Size was a deliberate consideration, since the group needed to be small enough to review each author's work weekly, and large enough to entertain potentially alternate opinions. Forming the work group were three faculty women with different but complementary talents, a commitment to professional excellence, and publishing histories indicating their capabilities for writing. They held different statuses on the faculty and were on different review timetables, so they were not in collateral competition in the school.

Group structure and process were both bounded by time. A contract for six weeks, subsequently extended to ten, was established, and the group met for a full day each week in an office away from the mainstream. The work pattern was to gather briefly in the morning to discuss goals, work separately for the bulk of the day, and reconvene to critique products. The expectation was that each member would present some written work for review.

Two significant time-related issues, punctuality and time use, affected group process and development and became apparent within the first few work sessions. Punctuality became an area of group concern to be tackled in relation to goals and purpose. Although tardiness never became a group norm, it came to be understood more clearly in relation to personal and professional obligations, as well as personal behavior. However, the group was never able to make punctuality a norm. As cohesiveness developed, the need to use the group as a source of support for the overall stresses of academic survival increased. The brief opening discussion period grew quickly to a whole morning. This use of time was acknowledged and debated. A group norm developed that allowed for flexibility based upon individual emotional need and the time-bounded task goals of the group. Each member assumed responsibility to carefully monitor time use. Monitoring centered on identifying issues of procrastination, creating realistic writing timetables, and determining the costs of using this worktime for ventilation and professional or emotional support.

One member entered the group with a considerably lower degree of commitment and interest in writing for publication. Time and effort devoted to her issues and attitudes was clearly at the expense of attention to other members' needs and writing efforts. The conflict was heightened by the limited time available for goal attainment. Reflective evaluation suggests that the effort served to create a high degree of cohesiveness, as well as to clarify the legitimacy and sincerity of the group's purpose, both of which are important issues to group survival.

Group outcomes can be described in terms of specific scholarly productivity and professional growth. The ten weeks' work resulted in a proposal and the completion of the related paper accepted for a special publication; completion of a book chapter; the development of an outline for a reader; two abstracts accepted for major social work symposia; final revisions of a paper and submission of it for publication review; and a draft of an article developed from one member's dissertation. In the area of professional growth, the regularity of meeting time and intensity of the work fostered an intellectual revitalization. Members developed attitudes of entitlement to time for scholarly writing as part of the normal work load.

Group commitment and affective stability have remained high. Group members recontracted on the original terms for two successive semesters, and subsequently for continued emotional support and stimulation for scholarly endeavor without structured work times. Productivity has fluctuated, and the critical relationship between structured time, support and the members' abilities to meet publishing expectations has been demonstrated.

Kathleen J. Pottick
Anne Currin Adams
Audrey Olsen Faulkner
Rutgers University
School of Social Work
New Brunswick, NJ

TIME LIMITED TRAINING FOR GROUP LEADERSHIP

It seems appropriate and perhaps necessary that some entry level group training be a part of every graduate social work program. Leadership experience, actual skill training, is expected to happen in the field placement. However, every social work student will not have the opportunity to learn this valuable skill within the traditional educational format.

This article describes a time-limited training program for group leadership that uses a group format for specific focused learning. The model of group work training presented here includes important theoretical conceptualizations where these skills can be practiced. Opportunity is available for immediate supervision and feedback on how the student has carried this out. All this takes place within an abbreviated time period, approximately twelve hours of a didactic/ experiential learning seminar followed by a supervised laboratory experience as a group leader for sixteen hours of a two and a half day weekend workshop.

Group Leadership Training Format

Use of a combination of cognitive and experiential training styles enables group leaders to become aware of and better deal with their feelings, stimulated by either the content matter or the intragroup dynamics and by immediate feedback. The knowledge and skills to meet the goals of good group leadership and the constraints of limited time are combined through a focused learning situation that closely parallels the actual leadership experience that the trainees will be expected to facilitate. The trainer models the appropriate leadership behavior as she/he guides the trainees through the two-day group experience. During this time, the content material that the trainees will use is explored and discussed. Fantasies and other group activities are experienced.

The training is divided into three phases: didactic, experiential, and skill development. In the didactic phase, a model of leadership intervention with its focus on mutual aid and a focus on work in the present experience and interaction is presented and discussed. This integrative approach is compared and contrasted with other frameworks of practice to help the trainees clarify for themselves what the group experience is expected to be. This is done by presenting expected issues that might arise during the workshop and by demon-

strating various leadership responses. The stages of group development to be expected, the dynamic characteristics of each stage, and
the "hoped for" leader focus are used to present a "minicourse" on
the life and flow of groups.

Phase II of the training is an experiential segment designed to increase the trainees' awareness of their own feelings around the
issues related to the content matter. For example, in training leaders
for a workshop in human sexuality, their attitudes are explored and
discussed while working through the same exercises, fantasies and
role-plays that the participants will be doing. Although this part is
heavily oriented toward experiential learning, the future leaders are
learning also on a cognitive level how to administer each task and
what responses they might expect and what they might do to cope
with this. By experiencing the participant's role, the anxiety of
beginning group leaders is reduced and the potential for empathy
with group members is increased.

The third phase of training involves skills development exercises
wherein future group leaders explore typical issues in content and
group process through the use of vignettes. Trainees have the opportunity to role-play leader behaviors in their own training sessions
and discuss and practice alternate reponses. An ending exercise
helps them to deal with the issues around termination by making
them aware of their own difficulties with separations and endings.

They are now deemed prepared for a supervised group leadership
assignment. The trainees as group leaders meet with their trainer for
"prep" periods prior to each group session. At the end of each day
there is time set aside for processing, questions, and sharing feelings
with other group leaders about what went on in their respective
groups. Ongoing supervision refines the application of principles. A
follow-up meeting during the succeeding week supports the learning
gained during the leadership experience. *(Edited.)*

Submitted by:
Barbara Dazzo
Clinical Social Worker
Somerset, NJ

PRACTICE QUIZ:
RECURRING ISSUES IN WORKING
WITH TIME LIMITED GROUPS:
FOUR VIGNETTES*

Practice issues that recur in groups can frequently be addressed by exploiting time limitations, when they exist. In the following vignettes, imagine yourself as the worker. How would you use the limited time factor to manage the issues (printed below in italics) in each instance?

Vignette 1—"Detox" Resistance

The setting is a short-term detoxification and alcoholic treatment center that provides five days of detoxification and treatment. The majority of the population is made up of chronic "skid-row" alcoholics placed in the group for three to five meetings. The focus of the group is on the "here and now" and the group is co-led by a staff member and a social work student.

Common issues include:

(a) Members are usually in the process of detoxification and thus, physically and emotionally unable to *fully relate* to the group process.
(b) Once the detoxification has progressed to an adequate level and the member no longer "feels sick," *denial* of the alcoholism problem becomes a factor.
(c) Generally, the alcoholic is referred on to another treatment program at the end of the five day detoxification period. This often is interpreted by the repeat client as a good reason to use the program as a "vacation" or as a means of getting off the street. He/she is thus, *not* easily *invested* in group process.

Vignette 2—Adolescent Anger

The setting was a large high school (4000 students) in an affluent suburban community. The group was structured to offer an opportunity to newly transferred-in students to deal with feelings, con-

---

*Based on material presented by graduate social work students Marcia Carlson, Margot Jedeikin, Brian Marvin and Judy Much.

cerns and questions relating to their transition into a highly competitive and organized system. All new sophomores, juniors and seniors were invited, in writing, to participate in the twelve meeting program. Seventeen accepted and participated in varying degrees with an average attendance of nine members. The solo worker was a second year graduate social work student.

While the group dealt with a range of issues relating to the difficulty of adolescents finding a way into a difficult new environment, an undercurrent of anger was a major constant in the early sessions. The anger, at first displaced in a variety of directions, when faced directly, became focused on parents who had made the decision to move, causing the uprooting and transplanting of the group members. It wasn't until this *anger* was *openly confronted and worked through,* at least partially, that the group could develop cohesion and begin to serve as a temporary reference group for the new students.

Vignette 3—Subgroup Competition

The group is made up of six graduate field-work students from two schools of social work placed for the semester in two adjacent teaching hospitals. There are students from both schools in each hospital. It is co-led by a social work staff member from each of the hospitals, neither of whom serves as field-work instructor to any of the group members. The co-leaders maintain a relatively non-directive leadership style.

Designed to meet for ninety minutes weekly for approximately twelve weeks, the group offers an opportunity for the student members to share experiences and growth as social work professionals and to learn about groups by being members of a group.

As of the fifth meeting they have not yet coalesced to select a specific thrust. A critical block to honest sharing and self-disclosure at this current point of group development appears to be the development of *competing hostile sub-groups* of four and two. The sub-groups also cross both school and agency lines and seem to represent differences in age and cultural background. To date, neither the student members nor the staff co-leaders have risked confronting the issue within the group. All members express discomfort with the situation which they recognize as responsible for the lack of group productivity. However, the discomfort and frustration apparently is not yet great enough to motivate the risk of confronting the issue directly.

Vignette 4—Couples Scapegoating

The group was designed as a closed, short-term (6 meetings) program for five pre-adoptive couples on the waiting list of a child welfare agency. The group purpose was viewed as providing: (a) information to the already screened couples and (b) a diagnostic opportunity different from the individual screening process. The group worker, a full-time staff member, selected the five couples from the waiting list pool including four new couples and one couple which was waiting for a second adoptive child. The "experienced" couple was included in anticipation of serving as a resource for the four "first-time" couples.

Although the resource couple was helpful in the first meetings in providing basic information and sharing significant experiences, they began to dominate the group discussion and to lecture the "first-timers" on how to "beat the agency system." The worker found herself unable to refocus and by the third and fourth meetings, the four "first-time" couples joined forces and confronted the monopolizers. They challenged with such communications as "What are you doing here? You already have a child." and "Are you manipulating us so that you can get a second child before we get a first?" Thus, the anticipated group resource couple turned into the *target* of *hostility* and *scapegoating* around which the group developed *questionable cohesion. (Edited.)*

Summarized by:
Joe Lassner, PhD, ACSW
School of Social Work
Loyola University of Chicago

AN EGO-ORIENTED, GOAL-DIRECTED,
SHORT-TERM TREATMENT MODEL
OF GROUPWORK WITH CANCER PATIENTS
AND THEIR FAMILIES

At the Michigan Cancer Foundation (MCF) in Detroit, Michigan (one of twenty (20) community cancer control agencies nationwide), a variety of time-limited groups apply the practice theories of ego psychology, crisis intervention, and stress management to a goal-directed problem-solving approach. Rehabilitation is the philosophical stance. All of this combined with the knowledge about how people cope with cancer, loss, and grief to develop the unique *gestalt* of their particular efforts. Specific elements include: validation of wellness, patient education, prevention, mutual aid, and ego-oriented goal-directed counseling.

The model focuses on the challenge of living with a life-threatening disease—cancer—and how one copes with the many realities that this disease imposes on the individual and the family structure. The purpose of this short-term group treatment for cancer patients and their families and friends is to provide an experience which will assist these individuals to better understand their cancer experience, to understand and to improve their coping skills, and to maximize their potential as they deal with a life-threatening illness.

A cancer experience, then, is a crisis situation which presents a variety of adaptive tasks which requires a combination or sequence of coping skills. It can best be understood as a stress event which may involve multiple crises, new dimensions of the original crisis, and may include the fear of crises yet to come. This, in turn, points to the vulnerability of the individual to ego dysfunction. It also provides a unique opportunity for the person to attain a higher level of functioning as coping skills are increased, as ego strengths are enhanced, and as one learns to cope with the threat of the crisis situation. An individual in crisis is, in most cases, an open person who is motivated to deal with her/his situation and thus is more amenable to social work intervention.

Since the individual's task becomes one of trying to return to a balance in ego functioning, the social worker's task is to facilitate this balance as well as to prevent the development of further dysfunctioning.

MCF Groups are closed short-term treatment groups which meet once a week for eight (8) weeks on a regularly scheduled basis.

The groups are led by Master's-prepared social workers with Bachelor's-prepared rehabilitation nurses as resource persons who attend the group for a maximum of three (3) sessions. The emphasis is on a *small group* experience, preferably six or seven members. The groups are thoroughly publicized through the full range of local media, direct mailing to all cancer patients and their families, and to identified professionals in the community. The groups are closed to new membership after the second session.

MCF offers the following groups: Men's/Women's Laryngectomy; Men's/Women's Ostomy; Cervical/Uterine; Mastectomy; Patient Group for All Diagnoses of Cancer; Laryngectomy Family and Friends, and All Diagnoses Families and Friends Group.

The content of the group process involves a variety of cancer-related issues which may encompass every aspect of the group members' lives, including physical, psychological, spiritual, vocational, sexual, financial and social components. For example: Attaining a better understanding of one's own individual cancer experience; physical management problems; loss, grief and death; the effect of body image alteration upon one's self concept, reactions of families and friends and how to deal with them, coping with the reality of returning to work, negotiating the health care system. The group ends on the note that the skills learned within the group are *transferrable to general use* outside of the group. Possible behavioral objectives related to the issues are articulated. This is correlated with individual goals stated in behavioral terms, actual "observables" used within the group process to evaluate the growth of each person.

Behavioral objectives deal with expression of feelings and concerns, disruption of one's body image and sexuality, realistic understanding of one's own diagnosis, treatment, and ongoing management, coping mechanisms for living with one's own cancer experience, one's own potential and redefinition of life goals, the health care system, expression of support, concern, and encouragement toward other group members.

The uniqueness of the MCF Groups is the blending of the following features during each session, thus creating special focus:

1. *Validation of One's Own Wellness.* Sharing experiences with others, as well as concerns and coping strategies, to obtain a baseline for one's own self-assessment; i.e., "I found out that I was a much stronger person than I had ever given myself

credit for''; and ''I found out that I wasn't crazy, but that I was trying to deal with a Hell of a disease.''

2. *Patient Education.* Understanding the medical aspects of one's cancer diagnosis, along with managing the physical aspects of the situation, further enhances one's control of many aspects of their experience. Seen as a technique of crisis intervention, patient teaching comes about through formal teaching, by nurses, social workers, community professionals and volunteers, informal teaching by the co-leaders, and through group teaching between members—all interwoven into the group process.

3. *Prevention.* MCF Groups use the group process to promote adaptive coping skills and to prevent maladaptive coping patterns from forming. For example: A woman in the Women's Laryngectomy Group was beginning to withdraw from friends and social contacts because she believed everyone was looking at her when she used her artificial device and they could see the scars from her radical neck surgery. Within the group, using role-playing, assertiveness training, processing of feelings, and guided group discussion, she was enabled gradually to return to her social contacts. She began to realize that by confronting her experience she was enabled to deal with it, thus, further withdrawal and isolation was prevented.

4. *Mutual Aid.* ''People helping people'' is reflected by such verbalizations as, ''I no longer feel alone'' and ''I have been inspired and encouraged not to give up by the support I have received from others in this group.''

5. *Ego-Oriented Goal-Directed Counseling.* The focus of the group depends on the identified goals of the group members and the specific areas that the group as a whole contracts to discuss. The commonality of cancer and the threat to life that this imposes are facilitative factors used to develop intimacy and to enhance group cohesion.

During the eight-week period, the skill of the leader is tested by the flow of time through the group. Initially, pre-diagnosis, diagnosis, surgery, and hospitalization are discussed, all reflecting a ''past'' orientation. During the middle phase, involving the most group time, there is the transition to ''here and now,'' how group members can best cope with their experiences. The ending phase focuses on actually identifying future goals and facilitating the group members' awareness of their own potential as people. "The group experience helped me to resolve some feelings and issues that I had about cancer. Now I can put them into a box and go on to other things, knowing that the cancer experience is here, but yet I have a lot of other living to do."

The task of the group leader is to maintain the focus during these discussions so that all can play their part in the problem-solving process.

The MCF Groups are evaluated by: (1) The group leader asking the group in various ways, on an ongoing basis, whether the group is meeting needs and how the group can be improved; (2) A Post-Session Reaction Sheet, which is a short one-page unstructured questionnaire; (3) An Evaluation Form with structured and unstructured questions; and (4) The assessment of individual goal attainment within the group process, using the behavioral objectives and the observables as guidelines for ongoing evaluation. *(Edited.)*

Submitted by:
Sarajane P. McNulty Schaefer, MSW, ACSW, CSW
Michigan Cancer Foundation
Detroit, Michigan

THE "CARING FOR YOUR AGING PARENT" GROUP

The "Caring for Your Aging Parent" group was organized by the social service department of a non-profit, 100-bed general hospital opened to the community at large. The idea arose from the author's years of experience working with adult children of aging parents (the "middle generation") who were facing major life situations of their own as well as their own parents' aging process and some of its difficulties (increased dependency, incontinency, issues of changing living situations, etc.). The emotional, physical and financial strains can be overwhelming and exhausting to family members. It was clear that many people shared similar concerns, fears and hopes, yet were experiencing their situation in general isolation. It was felt a group setting could help to lessen this sense of isolation and helplessness and at the same time, provide a forum for mutual problem-solving and sharing of coping strategies. The group setting also afforded an opportunity to share community resources, pragmatic information and some education around common concerns. The power of group members, of peers sharing similar concerns, was felt to be an extremely valuable resource and an effective medium. Group members would have a chance to decrease their feelings of guilt and diffuse their anger and at the same time increase their sense of support and control.

A general outline to help guide the group process was developed from existing literature and manuals relating to problems of grown children relating to their aging parents needs:

1. Introduction by group members of their own situation and an exploration of one's responsibility to one's parents.
2. What can one expect of their parents?
3. The aging process.
4. Our parents' expectations of us.
5. Discussion of area resources.
6. Review and termination.

The group structure was more formal in the beginning of the group. This time was used to assess/clarify group and individual goals.

The author gave a short (5-10 minute) talk the first night on the difficulty of reaching a balance between one's own needs and those of the aging parents. After a discussion period, members were asked to fill out a 3 x 5 card answering the following questions:

1. What can they reasonably expect from their parents?
2. What can their parents reasonably expect from them?   .
3. Their goals for the group?
4. What is one of their dreams/fantasies?

The cards provided a framework for subsequent nights' discussion.

The short term contract affected the depth of the members' interpersonal relationships with one another as well as affecting group and individual goals. This does not imply, however, that the relationships or the topics discussed remained at a superficial level. Quite the contrary. Topics were intense and members invested in sharing of themselves. The short term contract may have in fact enabled people to share as they knew they had only six weeks together. As the group developed, so did the sense of purpose and cohesion.

The short term nature of the group accelerated the group's progression through developmental stages. The group moved beyond the pre-affiliation stage through all the group stages. The pre-affiliation stage of the first group meeting involved ambivalency towards involvement, approach-avoidance behaviors and a greater reliance on distancing and role behaviors.

Subgroup formations were more apparent during the first meeting or two than during subsequent meetings. These appeared to be influenced by prior affiliations, one's socio-economic class, one's role in the home, one's situation, etc. By the fourth meeting there was a greater sense of intimacy in the group. Members were able to model appropriate ways of expressing anger as well as ventilating their feelings. Another indication of the increased intimacy was a shift in the group feeling more comfortable when acknowledging the benefits of nursing home care and a willingness to talk about their own individual struggles with that issue without "losing face" within the group.

Differentiation and separation stages were intermingled, because four members terminated at the fifth meeting. Separation was obviously a brief stage and yet one that underlied all previous weeks. The worker would remind the group each week where they were on the six week continuum, an element very important to time limited work. Problem sharing, clarification of feelings and support continued through the fifth and sixth sessions but group members also evaluated the group and their individual progress. Some comments about the group were "I gained a renewed sense of my own ability to cope"; "I liked being able to share ideas and feelings with others in similar situations"; "I enjoyed the frank discussion of problems and possible solutions." One woman shared at the last meeting that the group had helped her to decide to place her total care mother in a nursing home after caring for her for fifteen years with little family support and her mother's decompensating care needs.

The short term nature of the group undoubtedly left some conflicts and issues unresolved. Had the group gone longer, one might have focused more on conflict identification and resolution. Throughout the time-limited group sessions, the worker applied the following guidelines:

1. Being clear about group goals, limitation and priorities, not trying to "solve all or do all," thus avoiding frustration for both worker and group members alike.
2. Screening the applicants so that their needs and goals were

not beyond the scope of the group, thus remaining fair to the applicant, the group process, and to the group at large.

3. Using time to play a vital role in the group process, deliberation and purpose.
4. Helping members work within the time frame, intertwining function with the length of the group.
5. Because of the intensity of the group experience and its time-limited quality, being actively engaged "at all times," attentive and responsive to group members both individual and collectively.
6. Keeping the group in focus.
7. Sharing responsibility with the group members to help evaluate along the way and reach group goals.
8. Working towards the mutually-decided-upon group and individual goals within the time allotment.
9. Assessing as they arise whether the needs of group members can be met within the time frame of the group.
10. Addressing those unmet needs by referring group members elsewhere and/or assessing what avenues may best meet their needs.

The time limits on the group heightened the importance of keeping group members involved in their environment and community because their parents were to be reintegrated into the community very shortly.

The time limit on the group intensified the issue of member follow-up during the group for those members who missed one week as well as post-group follow-up. Responsibility of the worker for follow-up is intensified in time-limited social group work. Follow-up also helped with the evaluation of the long-term benefits of the short-term group work and aided future program development. *(Edited.)*

Submitted by:
Connie Morse McCaffrey, MSW
Exeter Hospital
Exeter, NH

Call for Papers

Contributions are invited for a special issue of *Social Work with Groups*. The special issue is to appear in the Fall of 1986 and will be devoted entirely to research in group work. Special guest editor will be Ronald A. Feldman of Washington University, St. Louis. Associate guest editors are Larry E. Davis (Washington University, St. Louis), Maeda Galinsky (University of North Carolina, Chapel Hill), Sheldon D. Rose (University of Wisconsin, Madison), Martin Sundel (University of Texas, Arlington), and James K. Whittaker (University of Washington, Seattle).

Consideration will be given to research reports, evaluations of group work programs, synthesis of research advances or methodological issues, operationalization of dependent and independent variables in group work practice or research, the study group developmental processes, and analyses of measurement issues or techniques. Original papers on any and all aspects of group work are welcome.

All manuscripts should conform to the requirements of manuscripts for *Social Work with Groups*. Papers can be submitted to the Special Editor for this issue at The George Warren Brown School of Social Work, Washington University, St. Louis, Missouri 63130. While deadline for submission is August 1, 1985, manuscripts will be welcome in advance of that date.

Call for Papers

A special issue of *Social Work with Groups* will focus on professional practice with task oriented work groups such as:

Teams

Treatment Conferences

Social Action Groups

Committees

Administrative and Fiduciary Groups

Councils and Interorganizational Groups

Papers should not exceed 20 double-spaced pages including references and abstract. Papers should be submitted *no later than October 1, 1985*, in triplicate, to either co-editor of the special issue. Inquiries and suggestions are welcome.

CO-EDITORS

Ronald W. Toseland
State University of New York—Albany
Rockefeller College of Public Affairs and Policy
School of Social Welfare
135 Western Avenue
Albany, NY 12222

Paul Ephross
University of Maryland at Baltimore
School of Social Work and Community Planning
525 West Redwood Street
Baltimore, MD 20201

DATE DUE

DHUW	MAR 3 1988		
AUG 6 1994			
DHUW	JUL 7	REC'D	
			DHUW MAY 24 ENT'D
SW MAY 1 0 1996 SW APR 4 1996			
DHUW APR 22 REC'D			
GAYLORD			PRINTED IN U.S.A.